DUDE,
You're Gonna Be a
DAD!

DUDE,
You're Gonna Be a
DAD!

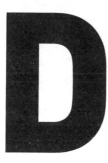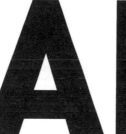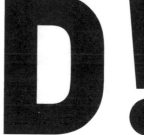

How to Get
(Both of You)
Through the
Next 9
Months

JOHN PFEIFFER

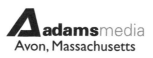

A adamsmedia
Avon, Massachusetts

dedication
To Kaitlyn, Lindsay, and Zoey:
Find out what you are passionate about, and chase it with
everything you've got. And know that we will always love you
more today than we did yesterday.

Published by
Adams Media, a division of F+W Media, Inc.
57 Littlefield Street, Avon, MA 02322. U.S.A.
www.adamsmedia.com

ISBN 10: 1-4405-0536-5
ISBN 13: 978-1-4405-0536-2
eISBN 10: 1-4405-0962-X
eISBN 13: 978-1-4405-0962-9

Printed in the United States of America.

10

Library of Congress Cataloging-in-Publication Data
available from the publisher.

This publication is designed to provide accurate and authoritative information
with regard to the subject matter covered. It is sold with the understanding that
the publisher is not engaged in rendering legal, accounting, or other professional advice. If legal advice or other expert assistance is required, the services of
a competent professional person should be sought.
—From a *Declaration of Principles* jointly adopted by a Committee of the
American Bar Association and a Committee of Publishers and Associations

Many of the designations used by manufacturers and sellers to distinguish their
product are claimed as trademarks. Where those designations appear in this
book and Adams Media was aware of a trademark claim, the designations have
been printed with initial capital letters.

This book is available at quantity discounts for bulk purchases.
For information, please call 1-800-289-0963.

CONTENTS

Part 3: Third Trimester

Acknowledgments

It is an honor and a privilege to be writing this book. I want to thank the many people in my life who obviously were overserved their share of patience. As long as I have this forum, and long after, I will thank my wife, Alana. Thanks for being so wonderful and supportive. I love you. To Kaitlyn, Lindsay, and Zoey: I want to send three heaping scoops of love, one for each of you. To Roy and Marie, Ken and Joan, the best grandparents our kids could have. To Marcia: may this effort do you proud. To Brendan at Adams Media, who made this project a reality. To Jenny, my devoted and skillful editor, who magically took my semicoherent manuscript and turned it into a book. To Michael Cunningham, whom I have never spoken to, but whose article gave me pause about my purpose and goals as a writer. Although great care was taken, any mistakes within are completely of my doing. Finally, to those who take the time to read this offering, I can only hope it proves in some way valuable to you, and somewhat entertaining as well.

Introduction
The Evolving Dude (er, Dad)

Pregnancy: the final frontier. It requires a total rewiring of your male thought process, which has been programmed since puberty to remind you to have sex responsibly and *not* impregnate your partner. So now that you're having sex to *try* to impregnate your partner, it's time to adjust to the idea of your life as a father.

As Dad-to-be, your primary job is to make sure Mom-to-be doesn't see red during this stressful time of emotional and physical upheaval for her, and to do your part to make the pregnancy as successful as possible.

This next stage—after conception—is all about research, planning, and making decisions. It's the way of nesting BMPs. What's that? Not familiar with the term? Your BMP is your "baby-making partner," that special someone you've chosen to embark on this journey with. And now that you have your partner, the challenge for you is to take an active part while all this gestating is going down. If you let it, the pregnancy game can swallow you up, leaving your BMP and her mother to make every decision. And you may think you're doing the right thing, being supportive and nodding your head in a north-and-south direction to every question thrown your way. But this can soon become a habit and before you know it, "Yes, dear, whatever you think," is your default setting. Until one day you wake up and realize you have a son named Percy and your wife is dressing him in a sailor suit. Your boy will already be off to a rough start—other babies will be plotting to steal little Percy's lunch money. If you let it go that far, it's extremely difficult to change things.

So the moral of the story is this: Give input right from the start. You need to carefully consider each decision. You have much to learn, grasshopper. Being informed and involved will make the process more fulfilling and less confusing, and of course it will help prevent the woman in your life from having to do all of the work. If creating a child takes two people, raising a child takes at least that many.

You need to stay on top of the ball and not get caught with your pants down—a position that's perfectly acceptable during the impregnation phase, but not so much when you're asked your opinion on critical issues like the color of the baby's room, or if and when Mommy is going back to work after baby arrives. You need to score a name for your child that you like but that still pleases Mom *and* all the grandparents. There's a lot being thrown at you and your BMP.

There are approximately 3,712 ways for a man to look stupid during the pregnancy, and I'm here to help you avoid (most of) them. Time is of the essence, and you need to prepare.

This urgency is caused by the fact that she's arming herself, as you read this, with knowledge about pregnancy and everything it entails. She is nose deep in books you would never spend two seconds reading. She will be filled with facts and figures, while you'll still be trying to figure out how Malcolm Gladwell gets his hair to look like that, and whether you could get away with that look.

If you don't step up to the plate, it will quickly become apparent that you know nothing, and after rolling her eyes and exchanging knowing looks with her girlfriends, your partner will start making decisions for you. This will quickly lead to a pattern in which she'll think that either you're stupid and incompetent or you just don't care about your child.

So although no man gets excited about getting a Brest Friend (it's not what you think) or about choosing the color of the car seat cover, your BMP is excited about these things, and that's what you need to care about.

So man up, get some knowledge of your own, and the entire process will go more smoothly for everyone. Arming yourself with this book was a step in the right direction. Now you have to finish reading it. If you do, you'll be happy because you'll know what's going on and what mistakes to avoid, and she'll be happy because her man cares so much about her and your soon-to-be-delivered boss.

Read, reflect, and evolve. It's not just about you anymore. It's time for you to turn into the leader of your pack. It's time for you to try on a new title: Daddy.

It is much easier to become a father than to be one.

—Kent Nerburn

To be any good at it, you'll have to grow and evolve, to change in ways that may not always be comfortable for you. As you experience these growing pains, you'll gain knowledge and the parent experience will get a little easier. As the great Jim Valvano once said: "Don't give up. Don't ever give up."

PART I

The First Trimester

The first trimester is a good time for both of you to mentally prepare yourselves and begin adjusting to your new lives as parents. Your BMP will feel changes in her body as pregnancy hormones begin to take effect. Her uterus will grow during this time, up to the size of a grapefruit, in preparation for the baby's growth. This little human comes complete with the DNA blueprint to form all of his or her body parts, from the halo atop her head all the way down to her toes. This baby will grow faster than your student loans: between day one and the ninth week of growth, the little fertilized embryo will grow to about an inch long. While every woman and every pregnancy is different, your BMP may begin to experience symptoms, including heartburn, headaches, mood swings, and morning sickness.

Dad, you will feel pretty good. Exactly the same, in fact. This is the first opportunity for you to begin to demonstrate that you are an engaged, motivated father. The best ways to do this will be to get informed, be supportive, and most of all, be patient. Oh, and if she gets a severe case of morning sickness, hold her hair while she gets sick.

CHAPTER 1

And We're Off

When the pregnancy test stick turns blue, the light to fatherhood goes green. It's something you've dreamed about most of your life. You and your buddies stayed up late, wearing your flowery pajamas, having tickle fights, and talking endlessly about your dreams of parenthood.

Or maybe not.

In any case, the time to prove yourself as a superior über-parent is fast approaching. If this book is in your hand, you're either an expectant father, or intentionally headed in that direction. You and your BMP are pushing the bobsled down the track and readying yourselves to hop in for a fast-and-furious ride that will be filled with thrills, chills, and of course, many, many spills.

When Conception Isn't a Piece of Cake

The pregnancy process is not as simple as those after-school specials make it out to be. Sometimes people have unprotected sex once and the magic takes place. Others try for

3

months on end with no results, only lots of frustration and disappointing moments.

Conception with Just the Two of You

If you're at the stage where you're *trying* to get pregnant, you need to keep your expectations realistic. You're expecting that little vixen to butter you up with a juicy steak, maybe some wine. As she refills your snifter, you put on your silk smoking jacket and take off your boxers, just to give her that little surprise when it's time. She's wearing your favorite lingerie and does a sexy striptease to get the mood right.

Guys, it's time to wake up. You're in her world now. Once a woman decides to get pregnant, there's no stopping her, and your sexual preferences aren't on the agenda. So, although you're 50 percent of the biological equation, you get about 10 percent input into the process.

How it works: Pretty much every month, she ovulates and her body gets ready to have a baby. So when your Barry White–influenced g-r-o-o-v-y sperm meets her egg, the shagadelic party in her uterus gets started. The good news is as a couple who intends to reproduce, you have a license to act like rabbits for a couple days each month. The bad news is that some factors can reduce your chances of getting pregnant and make the rabbit party end in frustration.

The bad news: If you're like most men, when she offers to give you oral, you're all, "Rock on, baby!" But oral stimulation actually decreases your pregnancy chances, because saliva kills your soldiers. Enough to make you cry, isn't it?

And that weird lubricant you bought from that shady store in the bad part of town? It also reduces your chances of conception, so put away the "liquid silk" you bought (or dig the receipt out of the trash and return it, if you kept that trench coat and fedora you used as your disguise).

Hot tubs and electric blankets? Sorry, those are on the no-fly list, too. Yes, guys, I am here to break the bad news to you: having sex to get pregnant isn't your ordinary, recreational nonpregnancy sex.

What to do: Your first course of action will be to have sex smarter, not harder (unless that's what you're into.) Ovulation kits will help your girl know when the egg is ready to launch and it's time to get your soldiers into battle. So whether it's noon on Tuesday or Sunday at 7 A.M., when the kit orders you to have sex, you must comply. It is strangely not as hot as it sounds. I tried to dress the ovulation kit up in a leather outfit and let it boss us around, but even that did nothing for me. It can become businesslike, especially when your partner asks you to hurry up and finish. Depending on the situation, you may even feel cheap and used for sex. Then you'll know why women get so mad about it when it happens to them.

Calling In the Professionals

After, oh, a year of this, if you're still not pregnant, then you'll want to move to the next step: medical assistance.

Depending on why your sperm and her egg aren't uniting, a doctor may prescribe one or more medications, such as Clomid (clomiphene), to help increase your chances of conception. An unwanted side effect may be that your BMP's hormone levels get driven off the charts. (Fire may actually shoot out of her eyes.) With luck, such medications and the repetition of well-timed attacks from your seed will yield the desired results. If not, your next step may be to embark on a long, strange trip to the infertility specialist. That's when things get weird. If you have to go this route, you'll have to be prepared—with an hour's notice—to give blood . . . and more. You'll be asked to fill up a cup with your most valuable fluid, and the only assistance will come from outdated "adult" materials that your friendly neighborhood fertility doc sorely needs to update. I hope you can avoid all of this and just work in conjunction with Mother Nature.

If you have to go down this road, be aware of the ramifications of the process. As each attempt at getting pregnant comes and goes, the stress and pressure to get "results" goes up accordingly. We are trained to be results oriented, and we are attempting to control Mother Nature. As frustrated as you may feel, your BMP will feel the same, only tenfold. As each failed attempt occurs, she likely takes the failure to get pregnant as a reflection on her. Now is the time for you to get "in the zone" for being at your supportive best. Light some candles, meditate, or even sniff some chamomile—do whatever you have to do to get ready to be there for your partner.

Finding Out

She suspects she's pregnant. She misses her period, or else she's charting her ovulation cycle and she knows you've got a good chance of getting good news. In a rush of excitement, she'll start the pregnancy testing game. Set aside $50 or more for this wonderful game. If she sends you to the store to pick up the pregnancy test kit, I recommend buying the economy pack.

Your BMP knows she can take a pregnancy test as soon as seven days after ovulation, but ten to twelve days is actually more accurate.

Your BMP knows she can take a pregnancy test as soon as seven days after ovulation, but ten to twelve days is actually more accurate. Trying to hold her off until twelve days will most likely require some rope, a couple of 2×4s, a tiger cage, and some ball bearings. On day number seven she'll take several tests. The most likely outcome will be a negative result, even if she really is pregnant.

Be advised, even if she gets a positive test, she will take several more tests just to be sure— hence the budgetary concerns. This means multiple trips to the pharmacy for you and lots of laser-guided urine attacks on testing sticks for your BMP. Don't be frustrated. This ritual opens the doorway to fatherhood. And don't discount the possibility of a physical celebration between the two of you.

If all goes well, at some point you'll get the good news: she's pregnant! Way to go, champ. Now you're feeling that unique emotion that bonds all first-time fathers together. It's best described as excitement tinged with a yellow streak of fear and a dash of nausea.

Your internal monologue asks if you're up to the challenge. "No worries," you think to yourself. "I have nine months before I need to be concerned about this. Besides, my beautiful mother-to-be will be taking care of most of it. My work here is done! Now back to conquering the entire Internet!"

Nope. Sorry, big fella. Operation Blue Cross was just the first step in the lifelong journey of parenthood. You may feel like king of the mountain at the moment, but time is a-wasting. Your bundle of joy is already growing, all the while working on a list of diabolical plots, from *Plan A: See How Many Diapers Parents Can Change in One Hour* to *Plan Z: Get Mom and Dad to Give Me ONE MILLION DOLLARS!*

You need to have counter-strategies and disaster-recovery plans in place—and it all starts with some questions for the dad-to-be: *What do babies eat? Do I need to start saving for college? What is the separation of responsibility between parents? Who is in charge of what? Do we need to apply to private school yet?* You need to provide for this little human.

You may hear how they "grow up so fast," but this is mostly a phrase used by old people who have lost their minds. It takes a lot of time and effort to get your kid launched. But fear not: with hard work, love, and a little help, you will be navigating this brand-new world without a problem.

Your Reaction

Your first reaction may be to pop the cork, open some wine, or shake a martini. Um, slow down there. Put the olives and vermouth away. Remember that the newly anointed mother of your child cannot drink alcohol. Unless she is kind enough to grant permission, you should refrain as a gesture of solidarity. You know, it's like you're saying, "Yep, we're in this thing together."

While you sip sparkling grape juice and reminisce about New Year's Eve when you were twelve, you'll probably wonder how long you have to get ready before the stork shows up. Traditionally, that number is forty weeks from the date of her last period. You'll get an "official" due date from the doctor based on information she gives him about her cycle, anything she knows about her ovulation, and other factors, but remember, it's only an estimate. In other words, don't get your firstborn's due date tattooed on your shoulder before the actual birth.

You may feel pressure begin to build as you realize that fatherhood is just around the corner. You may even experience pure, unadulterated fear. You will soon be a father and have all the responsibility that it entails. As you look down and realize your socks don't match and toilet paper is stuck to your shoe, you have a horrific vision of a baby depending on *you* for life's basic needs.

The joys of parents are secret, and so are their griefs and fears.
—Francis Bacon Sr.

Take a deep breath, and try to relax. You can do this. While it's certainly no walk in the park, less skilled parents are able to keep their child alive until age eighteen . . . or even longer! It may seem as if you're about to sacrifice all those things you used to enjoy for the sake of your family, but before you run away from home, just know that you're probably going to love being a dad more than you think. A strange phenomenon occurs when you have a whole bunch of stressful, exhausting days in a row and you think about changing your name to Juan Valdez and hopping the next plane to Parts Unknown, South America: your child will do something that makes it all seem worthwhile. Maybe it's a simple smile, or the way he greets you with a huge smile right when you arrive home from work. Maybe it's the first time you hear your child call you "Daddy." In ways both small and large, this child will affect you in ways you can't predict.

Her Reaction

Like most men most of the time, you'll be in touch with your feelings, but what about your BMP? She will most likely feel a hundred emotions at once. You are excited and thinking, "This is awesome." She is starting there, and then wondering how fat she'll get. Maybe she's feeling some fear at the thought of giving birth, hopeful that you are excited, and worried about labor pain . . . see what I mean? You can see how things are much different in BMP-World than for you and your simple caveman brain. In fact, she's already thinking . . . .

When and How Do We Spill the Beans?

About five weeks in, you'll start considering whether it's time to start telling everyone you know that you're having a baby. You and your BMP are feeling the love. You're about to bring a child into the world. The sun seems to shine a little brighter, and you're noticing things you've never seen before, like car seats, strollers, and how cute the clothes are in the infant section. Why have you never noticed these things before? As you find yourself idly thinking that you prefer the brown-checkered stroller to the green one, you're brimming with excitement, and it seems like the right time to start crafting a witty Tweet to your peeps announcing the creation of a life in 140 characters or less.

Sorry to keep reining you in, but please put down that iPhone. When it comes time for your big announcement, you can rest assured there will be "an app for that." But in the meantime you and your BMP need to come to an agreement on how to proceed before you go blabbing around town about the fruit of your lovemaking. Before you spill the beans, put the beer down for a second and listen: Miscarriages are hell. I've been there. The reason most couples wait until after the third month is that the chance of miscarriage plummets by quite a bit. If this happens, God forbid, you don't really want to have to go back and tell everyone about this very personal and very painful thing that just happened.

So the old-school method is to wait until around weeks 8 to 12, when the mathematical chances for miscarriage go down significantly. The actual chance of miscarriage at this point in the pregnancy is somewhere in the neighborhood of 5 percent, depending on what study you're looking at. Most guys say to themselves, "Great! We'll do it week 12! Now let's go look at a flat-screen TV for Junior's room." But a quick scan of pregnant women's websites will tell you that mothers today don't consider the decision so black-and-white. It's difficult for the two of you, who are so excited about this great news, to contain yourselves and keep from accidentally having a slip of the tongue. You may give it away accidentally from something as simple as cutting out a magazine article on pregnancy and leaving it lying on the counter. So, my best advice is to make a plan on which you both can agree about when to break the news, and keep it to yourself until then.

When to Tell

After conversing with a number of pregnancy veterans, I put together this plan for your consideration:

First Month

Keep it on the down low (unless that means what my wife told me Oprah said it means—then forget I used this phrasing!). The two of you can exchange knowing glances and have your own little secret all to yourselves. Many people will go ahead and let their close family know, but be warned: some grandparents-to-be can be, well, *intense*. They can pick a name, buy clothes for the baby, and help her apply to college all while you're still looking at the plus sign on the pregnancy-test stick. The whole thing escalates to a new level. Just make sure the grandparents know before the public at large. If they're the last to know, they may never forgive you, and surely you'll need them to help out in the future.

Second Month

Trial and error has proven the best way to go here. You can each tell one friend, as friends can share in your excitement, and you'll have someone new to discuss this grand news with. Yes, this is more for her benefit, as most guys will exchange fist bumps and then get back to sports or the stock market.

Third Month

It's about time to release the hounds. Tweet, Facebook, e-mail, go for it all, as long as you both agree to it. If you want to, have a baby shower . . . more on that later. But back to some of the more creative methods to alert friends and family of your BMP's condition:

1. Feeling nostalgic? Plaster "Baby on Board" stickers all over your house and car.
2. Give your parents and/or in-laws a "World's #1 Grandparent" T-shirt, and watch them smile.
3. Even the dimmest family members will get it when you ply them with copies of the ultrasound photo; e-mail them the website link or wrap up a printout in a gift box.

There is also the matter of the family hierarchy, something you'll need to consider to prevent hurt feelings on the part of friends or family. Let's say that during a chance meeting at the mall you blurt out the good news to a friend you happen to run into. This seems harmless, because it came from the excitement you've been feeling. Right? Unfortunately, this is incorrect. Let's say this was a lesser friend, who tells one of your BMP's best friends over the phone two weeks later. Guess who the bad guy is? This example can be directly applied to all family. If you happen to be eating dinner with an aunt who's in town for work, and you informed her before your own sister . . . there's going to be drama. Hurt feelings and flaring tempers ensue. Relatives in Atlanta call in to *The Bert Show* to tell much of the Southeast how inconsiderate you are. Perhaps this is why most people seem to favor a simple, drama-free strategy such as telling future grandparents first, and sending out a mass e-mail of the ultrasound to everyone else. It might seem less personal than spreading the news to friends and family one by one, but it's simple and effective. You're off the hook.

Time to Talk:
Conquering Fears, Being Supportive,
and When to Say Nothing

Men are men. This simple and absurd statement can be exhaustively analyzed until your head spins, and I plan to do just that. Men, you and I are simply men: the stereotypical man. Some of the expectations that come with being the stereotypical man? He is indestructible, is weakened only by kryptonite, can fly, and is a poor communicator.

We tend to keep things, such as problems or concerns we're having, to ourselves. Our role upon entering manhood initiation was to carry all burdens that were given to us and never discuss our feelings. Ever. So, because communication is such an important part of any adult relationship, especially including ones involving a baby, we need some solid help from the women in our lives.

Dads Unite!

Staying informed is one thing women as a whole execute better than we do. They organize and analyze. They have so much information available to and targeted at them, it would be hard for any female with an Internet connection not to be a well-informed pregnant lady. But I was thinking of what old dads (like me) would tell a newly minted pregnant mother (your BMP) about how to help the newest daddy on the block (you) during this time of adjustment for everyone. See if you can get her to read this section. Try leaving the book open on her pillow or telling her you want to swap pregnancy books with her. While you're fake-reading her book, watch her read this one and see her reaction. If this section gets you into trouble, you can always claim you haven't read this far and disagree with everything I've written.

Better yet, use this as an excuse to discuss some of these things that might not be easily covered over the course of normal day-to-day conversation. (It's quite possible I'm pulling some sort of triple-reverse-psychology trick on you, and I'm going to tell you things for your own good.)

For the Mom-to-Be . . .

Here are some things you may have trouble saying to your BMP; I'm going to say them for you:

He Feels Left Out in the Cold

The whole baby thing is taking place inside the mother, and physically, she's undergoing the most changes. But with everything so focused on Mommy, Dad sometimes can feel like the sperm donation was the key part for him to play. Doctor's visits, admiring the baby bump—of course that's where most of the focus will be. But many of these items do not directly involve your man, and they're not natural activities that he's going to dive right into. It can all add up to a dad who isn't feeling connected to the baby right up through the whole birth process.

So BMPs, encourage Dad-to-be to make himself heard, and whether it feels natural or not, to get in there and participate. Ask him to vote for yellow over green for the nursery, and get him to read this and other pregnancy books, go to birthing class, and do whatever it takes to keep him from being swept off the map. It's an adjustment for him, but with so much of the focus being placed on the baby, and rightfully so, new dads are sometimes lost in the shuffle and disengage from the process like Maverick in *Top Gun*.

This Pregnant Woman Is Difficult to Deal With

There, I said it. And I'm not taking it back. Dealing with a pregnant woman can be like dealing with an unhappy person with multiple-personality disorder. It seems like there are many personalities in there and we can't switch gears fast enough to keep up. To hang tough, your guy needs to know that the woman he loves is in there somewhere. How can you show that? The easiest answer is to do something that the two of you used to do together. But don't be afraid to break away from the herd. You two are beginning a totally new type of relationship, so you may want to dream up a new activity accordingly. Go have dinner and declare the conversation to be baby-free. Although most people look at children as the glue to a family, it's actually a strong relationship between the parents that matters most. Keep up the required maintenance on your relationship, and make sure all the parts of the relationship are running smoothly. (Yes, I just compared your relationship to cars.) Point your man to websites dedicated to pregnant women, where he'll discover useful information (as well as how the idea that pregnant women are allowed to say or ask just about anything from us gets perpetuated).

He Gets the Blues Too

Ladies, if you've done your homework, you know the risk of depression that women can face around pregnancy and parenthood. Men are at risk as well. A new study shows that up to 15 percent of men suffer from postpartum depression. And that's only the number of wimps who are actually willing to admit it. Between the emotional and financial stress and friends and family focusing on the glowing mom or the arriving baby, Dad is out of the spotlight. He is treated like an old dog; just throw him a few bones of attention and he'll lie down contentedly for a nap. But when he gets the "just a sperm donor" treatment, it's a tough adjustment.

Let's not forget that post-birth depression is not only for women. Finally, something we can share! Unfortunately, after Junior comes home, both Mom and Dad can feel overloaded, unsure, and exhausted. Despite what the pharmaceutical industry says, no magic pill can make it pass (if you disagree, ignore my advice and go see a doctor). But talking it out (I know, we men hate to do this) and trying to stay as rested and healthy as possible are good first lines of defense.

Share with Your Man

A note to women: he's not used to sharing you. He's used to getting most of your love and attention, and whenever possible, a little extra something-something from you. On a personal level, he wants to know he's still your special guy. He is losing your attention pre-birth, and he's sure to lose it post-birth. So be creative, and spend some time just with him. Give him a week where he's the only one who gets to touch the baby bump. Be flexible and take him to Vegas. Okay, maybe that's going too far. But you need to work together to keep each other happy.

He's worried because he knows that the new family member not only takes away some of your time and attention but also affects your sex life.

Please take note: sex is very important to most men. Can this be stressed enough? Don't get me wrong; your man will enjoy having a baby and will be excited. It's just that part of his relationship with you has this most enjoyable special form of interaction. So please don't forget about it, because he didn't.

Give Me a T!

All of those things that pregnant women need to do before their guilt overwhelms them—like eat healthier and exercise? Make him go along with you. Everything is easier with a friend, and if you and your man are creating a child together, you at least qualify as friends, and will remain so. Oh, and you're giving me a T, as in T-E-A-M, because you're in this together and need to help each other out. You will need each other to play different roles through this new challenge. Some days you'll need to motivate each other, some days you'll need to complain to each other, and some days you'll just need to play straight up "boss and secretary" with each other. But whatever each day brings, you'll always need each other.

Make Him Talk

I can't believe I'm saying this after all those times when I didn't feel like talking about something. But it has to be done. Since guys don't call each other up and chit-chat about how being a father makes them *feel* or about their *fears* (just so you know, we have none), it's up to you, a VIP BMP, to pull this stuff out of your man and make him discuss it.

Because hey, he's got worries too, or at least he will when he stops and realizes what having a baby means to your lives. So unless you have the rare man who begins a conversation with, "Hey, honey, I have some concerns about what having a baby together will mean to our relationship and our lives together," he may need you to get the ball rolling.

Be Patient: Remember That He Doesn't Always Plan Things Out

This may be an understatement. Most men certainly don't think about our plan, and then think again about our plan, and then plan to further plan. Unlike the baby, some of his thoughts and last-second plans are poorly conceived. You, the BMP, may have read three articles and changed your opinion on an issue twice before you ask him. He usually thinks for about two to three seconds, and gives you his best guess. So please work with him on these conversations and try to avoid ambushing him with questions like, "What will we do if our new daughter has trouble making friends with other children?" Ummm, he doesn't know. And he hasn't thought about it, but it doesn't mean he doesn't care. If this rule seems to work in the child arena, test it out in other parts of the relationship as well.

Change He Can Believe In

Dads are committed to being good parents, but in today's world it can be difficult to reconcile his mental image of himself as a strong, virile man while he's pushing a stroller decorated with bunnies, carrying a pink diaper bag, and holding the door open for other fathers on his way into baby yoga class. It can make him feel slightly less than manly, and all of these activities can also make him late for his facial and body waxing. So while he needs to work on being more sensitive to the myriad changes you're experiencing, his big lumbering male ego will need a tune-up as well.

Promises, Promises

Please, please let us know that while the frequency may be greatly reduced, there will still be post-pregnancy time for you to feed him buffalo wings while dressing suggestively and painting his toenails while he watches football. (Wait, maybe I'm all alone on toenail painting.) But you can work something out to ensure that you do fun and special things together after Junior becomes part of the family. Leave your man a note with your perfume on it, with only a date, and no explanation. Send a calendar reminder to his e-mail or electronic calendar that says, "Human Resources Training: Sexual Harassment," and then show him how to break all the policies in the employee handbook. This might just start a playful back and forth that will keep the relationship fun for everyone.

Ok. Thanks for taking the time to hear us out. Off you go, and let Dad back in the saddle. . . . Is that you? Glad you're back. Now let's get to it.

Get Into Bondage—No, Really

Here's the good news: it's time for some bondage. Don't worry, your BMP will be thrilled you're so into it, and it's been proven to be good for your unborn child. Here's the bad news: we aren't talking about doing strange things in the bedroom with fuzzy purple handcuffs; we're talking about bonding with your BMP and your unborn child. For guys, bonding with an unborn child can be difficult, especially in the first few months, when you can't see any visible signs that the child exists.

Bonding with your woman should be easy enough. You've already explored one form of bonding to get here. But now it's time to bond in more creative, yet less orgasmic ways.

Talk about what these life changes are going to mean for both of you. Discuss plans for your child after her birth. Make it clear to your BMP that you still expect a hot meal and foot rub upon your arrival home from work. These are the important things that will ease the changes that are sure to happen.

Building a relationship with your unseen child can feel a little strange. Suggested methods include massaging your BMP's belly and talking to your creation. Diagram football plays on your BMP's belly while giving a full explanation. Listen to music for a few minutes each day with your child. Doctors recommend classical, but who knows? If you like Barry Manilow, who's to say your child won't start kicking to "Mandy"?

If it feels slightly unnatural to stare into your BMP's navel and tell the fuzz lingering in there how your day went, don't worry. It's all part of the birthing process. Just come up with something you can accept that will begin forming that bond between you and your child. (Do I have any suggestions? I thought you'd never ask!)

Here are a few more concrete activities that will help you build that bond:

- **Doctor's visits.** There are a lot of these, but try to think of them as time you're taking together to check on Junior's health, and to stay informed about what's going on. See Chapter 3 for more about this.

- **Ultrasound.** This is a major bonding moment for a lot of people. You will confirm that all the fingers and toes are there, and learn the sex of your child, if you desire. If you really want some fun, check around the area to see if 3-D ultrasound is available. Reports are that the details are stunning—you can see exactly what your child is doing in there and what he looks like.

- **Discussing Junior's future.** So it seems farfetched to talk about where your baby may attend college, but a nice discussion of your child's future is allowed to drift into what might be referred to as "slightly optimistic" territory. Dream a little dream together, and let it bring you closer together emotionally. If it does the same physically, so much the better.

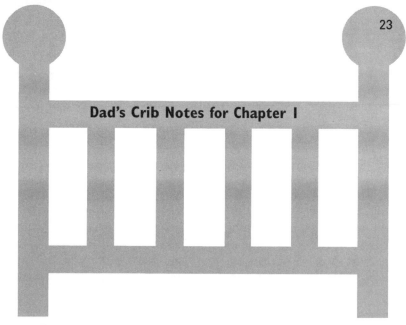

Dad's Crib Notes for Chapter 1

- Conception isn't always as easy as those after-school specials made it out to be.
- Be ready to purchase a 12-pack of pregnancy tests. She'll want to make sure, and then check it several more times. Go ahead and be excited!
- You will both be full of hope—and fear. Now is the time to man up and talk about this with you partner.
- Don't worry; you can't see it now, but you're going to love being a dad.
- Traditionally, you do not spread the news about the pregnancy until around week 12. But the two of you should discuss just exactly how you want to do it.
- There is a lot of information concerning the challenges women face during pregnancy, but men, we have our own things going on.
- Trying to bond with your unborn child will seem strange at first, especially because you can't see her, but why not try?

CHAPTER 2

Taking Care of Her

Your BMP is having to go through a lot of changes. Her hard-won figure will soon be transformed. Her mobility will decrease. She may experience constant nausea. She's suffering all of this in the name of having a baby with you. So your best possible move is to attempt to make her pregnancy easier by any means. Find out things she has to deal with in her everyday life that you can take off her hands, even if it means a little extra effort on your part. Be considerate of things she can no longer do all the time. If she's having troubles with morning sickness, keep crackers and ginger ale in all parts of the house. Finally, let her know you love her. Plan a good old-fashioned date night, complete with flowers and some well-thought-out plans. It might be a fun time to relive some of those old memories.

Handling the Hormones

I hate to stereotype, but it requires so much less thought. So if the following description doesn't jibe with your experience, I apologize in advance. The implantation of the egg into her uterus causes the production of hCG (or beta hCG), the pregnancy hormone. This causes production of estrogen and progesterone. These hormones are quite necessary for the development of the baby, but like steroids and unprotected sex, they have side effects. As production of the hormones continues, the levels in her body begin to increase. During weeks 5, 6, and 7, pregnancy hormones start making your BMP crazy. Like DEFCON 1 crazy. Typical symptoms include nausea, fatigue, and tender nipples, plus urinating more than your grandfather.

The funny thing is, *your* hormone levels are changing as well. According to recent research, your levels of cortisol, the fight-or-flight hormone, surge and spike about six weeks after you get the news about the pregnancy. Also, about three weeks before birth, your level of testosterone reduces by nearly one-third. So the baby is changing your woman and making you want to run away crying at the same time. If another guy challenged your manhood, you would be more likely to engage him in a slap fight or maybe a runway duel, à la *Zoolander*. It's no wonder new parents don't feel like themselves, because of all those changes in their lives and their bodies. Strap yourself in and get ready for the only thing you know for sure: changes are coming your way.

You Versus the Hormones

You versus the hormones is like Spinks versus Tyson, Joe versus the Volcano, and Tiger versus monogamy. You have no chance. The pregnancy hormones are just too strong. They make her emotions change, and they make her body change. Lots of regular foods she used to enjoy might make her react as if you just cut loose some mighty Taco Bell–driven wind. Her moods may become as unpredictable as a roulette wheel, and you'll have similar odds at predicting them. Fatigue becomes a major issue for her, and her bedtime and dinnertime may start to coincide with one another. But on a positive note, her all-day sickness (we're starting a campaign to rename "morning sickness") may show some signs of slowing down, although for many women it rages on into the second trimester before subsiding. Constipation and flatulence, gifts from your unborn angel, may become significant at these times. Just pretend you're back in freshman year of college with a roommate who has rapidly gained weight, farts all the time, and sleeps a lot. But there is one important difference. The extra bra size she has gained has you thinking this pregnancy may have some benefits after all.

Morning Sickness: Like a Really Long Hangover

Before you cook up your extra-onion cheesesteaks for dinner, you should know that morning sickness can be a 24-hour event, so she may puke on your briefcase just from the smell. Over half of all pregnant women go through morning sickness, which usually takes on the form of nausea and vomiting. Symptoms begin in the ballpark of week 6, and mercifully, they seem to end somewhere around week 12. A very select group of lucky women feel like crap all the way until delivery. But you don't have to worry, because you feel fine, right? Um, no! Of course you're concerned about your BMP, though there's usually nothing to worry about. Increased hormones in her body cause this cureless ailment, and as the hormones settle down, so will the morning sickness.

About one in every 250 women suffers from extreme morning sickness, called hyperemesis gravidarum, which often requires hospitalization.

About one in every 250 women suffers from extreme morning sickness, called hyperemesis gravidarum, which often requires hospitalization. It is an extreme form of morning sickness in which the nausea is severe, and a pregnant woman's inability to keep food and liquids down begins to actually cause weight loss. Signs will also include those of dehydration—severe thirst and dry cracked lips—as her body craves sustenance.

So what can you, the man guilty of *two* major offenses— you got her pregnant, and you feel fine—do to help improve the situation? Here are some of the basics:

1. Eat smaller, more frequent meals with her. Do more of the meal planning.
2. Avoid meals with strong smells (Chinese, anyone?) and very spicy dishes.

3. Keep lemons and ginger around. Smelling lemon can help reduce nausea, and eating ginger does the same. (Try crystallized ginger or ginger candy.) Keep salty chips or crackers around; they may dull the symptoms enough to allow her to eat a meal.

4. Make sure she has crackers and ginger ale near her bed at all times. Get her something to keep them in. Yes, you are being domesticated.

5. Stock the kitchen with all kinds of soothing bland foods like chicken noodle soup and potatoes.

6. Even though it will be the last thing she wants to do, encourage her to exercise. Walking is always good, and many doctors actually think swimming is the best because there is no impact on the joints.

7. Remind her not to lie down after eating. It can worsen the symptoms.

8. Encourage her not to skip meals, even when she feels lousy. Having a completely empty stomach can bring on the nausea. Skipping meals will usually make her feel even worse

9. Don't start a surprise tickle fight. It could be bad for your long-term health when your BMP either beats you to a pulp or "accidentally" vomits on you.

10. Don't let your partner enter a hot-dog-eating contest—or do anything resembling gorging if the nausea subsides for a little while.

Depending on how serious and frequent her morning sickness is, she may not be able to cook very often, so it's time to step outside your cooking comfort zone and find something else besides pizza and microwave food to prepare. You should be able to come up with a few specialties that you can prepare acceptably well. Do I expect you to make "preggie pops" in an assortment of pastel colors? No. I think that's going too far. But see what you can do to make her life easier.

Chores, Daddy Style

At the beginning, you were just so glad to be pregnant. As your little science project grew, your BMP began to wear down, up to the point where if she was eating at all, she was elbowing seniors out of the way at their favorite Early Bird Special spot so she could get to bed by 6 P.M.

In other words, your woman will be exhausted most days, especially if she's maintained gainful employment. At this point, it's time for you to start to pitch in. By pitching in, I mean doing more than telling her the buzzer on the dryer went off, or mentioning that the place looks so good you've decided to have poker night at your house.

The kind of man who thinks that helping with the dishes is beneath him will also think that helping with the baby is beneath him, and then he certainly is not going to be a very successful father.
—Eleanor Roosevelt

Men in general show support and affection by providing financially for their families. These men may attempt to help by bringing in cleaning services to knock out those things called chores. But women don't always take kindly to having strangers invade their home. Besides, many times you have these invasive (and expensive) strangers come in to clean, only to find they have done everything wrong in the eyes of your significant other. The best, but most unattractive, solution may be to show support with your actions, even if this includes scrubbing toilets and doing the laundry.

If you can pull off these chores with a smile, just know you will be in select company. (Remember Alice on *The Brady Bunch*? Cook, clean, do laundry? Just be careful not to enter Greg's room without knocking first. He's a teenage boy, after all.)

Helping Her Appreciate Her New Body (Lovin' the Curves)

Of all the changes Junior will bring to your schedule, social life, financial life, and sex life, it's the physical changes to your BMP that are starting to be most obvious now. Quite a few changes are going on, both inside and out. Let's take a moment to consider some of them. Yes, Sparky, I know: breast enlargement is one of them.

1. Belly. Somewhere around week 12, the baby begins to pooch out. Between months 2 and 3, her uterus will have grown to her belly button. By the end of the whole shooting match, that little miracle will have stretched things out up toward her rib cage.
2. Breasts. I will attempt to keep this section purely as it pertains to the gestation of your future child. Her breasts are preparing to produce milk for the baby. Estrogen, among other hormones, is working to increase the glands that produce this nutritious

liquid. During pregnancy, these changes can often lead to breast enlargement (see, I'm biting my tongue). Her breasts may feel slightly firm, and are often tender (. . . trying to hold back). Your partner may need a bigger bra as this growth progresses. Oh, for God's sake, let the puppies breathe!

3. Heart. Okay, I'm back. Sorry for that unnecessary outburst. Because of the future child taking up residence in Hotel Uterus, your BMP's blood supply will increase by one-third to one-half by the end of her pregnancy. In turn, her heart has to work harder to move this blood around. Her heartbeat can change from a usual resting rate of about 70 beats per minute to a resting pace of between 80 to 90 beats per minute. Keep this in mind when you're out for your daily twenty-miler with your BMP. She may not be able to keep up with her usual pace.

4. Gastrointestinal system. Those good old hormones are at it again. Some of the same hormones that are vital to maintaining a healthy pregnancy can also cause nausea and vomiting, along with other GI problems. If the breast enlargement section got you all hot and bothered, here's the antidote: belching, constipation, and increased flatulence are common during pregnancy. How's that for a cold shower?

5. Skin. The ever-present hormones can cause her skin to show brown patches as additional melanin is produced. There are even special rashes only pregnant women experience.

6. Joints and muscles. Your BMP's joints and muscles even change, to allow for the increased size of her uterus. Joints and ligaments loosen and stretch, and

while this is a wonderful thing for a growing baby who wishes to expand his home, it usually presents itself in the form of backaches for Mom and puts her at greater risk for tears and sprains.

So love her body, whatever the shape or size. Encourage her. Touch her with familiarity, whether it's with a gentle neck rub or holding her hand at the mall. The bottom line is that you want to communicate to her your feelings for her haven't changed or wavered no matter what her shape is at the moment. All you can hope for is that she'll return the favor as you slowly lose your figure, hair, and all sense of style.

Managing Weight Gain

Your BMP is going to gain weight. Another human is trapped in there, after all. So there's some truth to the saying that she's eating for two. But you, on the other hand, are not, so don't act like it. Whether you're eating for one or two, all bodies actually prefer a healthy diet to a steady stream of chicken wings.

You may be picturing her being all healthy while you continue to plow through a plate of cheese fries. I don't recommend it. It would feel like watching your friends accidentally stumble into a free all-you-can-drink event sponsored by the Swedish Bikini All-Stars on the night when you're the designated driver. So be considerate and behave around her. Moderation in your drinking, especially if it was something she enjoyed before pregnancy, is the prudent course. If the impregnation magic happened after a night of partying, don't pull out the "It reminds me of our night together and our child's conception" speech. She ain't buying it, no matter how great your sales skills. Playing the game this way may even earn you a couple of guilt-free nights out, with your BMP's blessing. The key word is *might*.

As for smokes, give them up. It's for your own good—and your baby's. Secondhand smoke will have your child sounding like a truck driver and rebuilding carburetors before his or her third birthday, not to mention all the other health conditions it can cause or worsen.

As your BMP gains weight with the growth of your seed, you may also gain weight. Don't give us the research about "sympathy weight." Do something good for yourself and eat healthfully with her.

Pickles and Ice Cream

If you watch enough movies, you'll see a poor father-to-be sent out in the middle of the night because his pregnant wife craves something. You've seen it before, right? The clock shows 2 A.M. and she shakes the poor boy awake. Invariably, she tells him that he needs to run to the store right now for some bizarre combination of foods. The guy, of course, simply cannot say no to her because she's pregnant. Much humor ensues.

It's true. Many report that their BMPs craved food from a certain restaurant. Some claim their partners wanted salty foods, while others say it was an ice cream sundae that was in such demand. The medical field hasn't conclusively documented the reasons for these stereotypical cravings. Their theories remain just that. As any man who has been through the process will tell you, it's probably best just to get her what she wants, when she wants it, if humanly possible.

Despite the hype, I've never been asked to run to the store at midnight for pickles and ice cream. Except for that one time in college . . . but nobody was pregnant.

Despite the hype, I've never been asked to run to the store at midnight for pickles and ice cream. Except for that one time in college . . . but nobody was pregnant.

Pregnancy Massage

It's time for the two of you to reconnect. I understand that your secret weapon is the art of seductive massage. I further understand that taking this weapon of mass seduction away from you is like sending a gladiator into the ring without his sword. But alas, I need to de-sword you. Don't try to play amateur masseur here. Incorrect massage can trigger contractions. Aromatherapy can also cause problems. Find a massage therapist who is specially trained in massaging pregnant women, and give your BMP a gift certificate.

Or better still, take the time to learn what massages you can safely give (ask her doctor). With all of the remodeling going on, she's likely to be sore. By likely, I mean 100 percent of pregnant women report feeling this way. Besides, what better way for you two to relax together?

Pregnancy Sex

Having sex once she's pregnant is overkill. Just kidding! It's not as easy as it was, though. Between your feeling strange about the whole "sex while pregnant" situation and everything she's got going on in there, it can get quite complicated when it comes to celebrating your love with your lover.

Her hormone count is higher than the number of Brett Favre comebacks (but not by much!), so be ready for anything, from multiple orgasms to weeping. As for where she falls on the sleep-all-the-time/sex-all-the-time scale, that can actually change during a commercial break, so be ready to miss the second half of *Grey's Anatomy* for unexpected sex.

Depending on your luck, your BMP won't look any different for three or four months, and during months four through six, if you blink really fast you can convince yourself she still doesn't look any different. With your doctor's assurance in hand that you can't hurt the baby (please direct real questions about this issue to your doctor), you can let your manly instincts take over. Now it's business as usual in the bedroom and without worries about getting her pregnant, because you're already there!

But at some point, there's no denying it: she's pregnant and you can really tell. As for the prospect of having relations with a very pregnant woman, I say you go all in. Presumably you love this person, and as long as your doc gives you the thumbs-up, it's all good. Don't underestimate the fact that once the little angel has arrived, you'll be exhausted for the next twelve months or more, and the energy you used to put into planning a sexy rendezvous will be gone. Instead of spending your free time on frivolous things like your hobbies and the laundry, your waking moments will be consumed with thoughts of a nap. Nap in the car, nap in the afternoon, spot-nap on the Burger King counter while waiting for order #123. Once that bundle of joy and tears arrives, you will take sleep wherever and whenever you can get it. By now you should be starting to get the point. Your sex life, among other things, will be drastically affected, and you two need to enjoy each other while your time and energy permits. So *why are you still reading*? Go get her!

Exercise During Pregnancy

Let's face it. In today's world of fifty-hour workweeks and long commutes, we all need some exercise. But it's especially important for your BMP to get regular exercise during her pregnancy. What are the benefits? More energy, sounder sleep, increased muscle strength, and reduction of various pregnancy symptoms, as well as the benefit of bouncing back into shape faster post-pregnancy than if she doesn't exercise.

If she's already exercising regularly, she'll probably be able to continue her routine. Of course, all exercise programs need to be cleared with her doctor first. If she isn't already active, it's unlikely that she'll be encouraged to start an intensive exercise program, but mild exercise, like walking, can still benefit your BMP. Pregnant women may also benefit from yoga classes specifically targeted toward them. Don't miss the opportunity to skip working out your already perfect pectorals to do a workout with her. She will appreciate the support, I promise! (Did I mention that you need to consult your real doctor first?)

Here's a wild idea: if you aren't exercising already, why don't you do the same? It can only help people on the street be able to tell definitively which one of you is pregnant.

Maternity Clothes

Forget your dog, maternity clothes are a man's real best friend. What man doesn't love special shopping trips where you purchase clothes you know for a fact will only be good for a few months? Adding to the fun is the fact that many maternity clothing stores are very proud of their clothes. You can tell by the amount they overcharge you.

The good news is that you now have evidence that she wasn't just faking it for the last few months to turn you into her personal slave. Now the bad news: she's going to need a whole new wardrobe. If you're lucky, you can beg, borrow, or steal what salvageable "gently used" maternity clothes you can from friends and family to minimize the financial impact. Otherwise, you're going to spend a mortgage payment on clothes. One more tip: if she asks your opinion when trying on clothes, go neutral.

> One more tip: if she asks your opinion when trying on clothes, go neutral.

A quick note, though: don't get rid of these clothes if you plan to have more children, or if you plan to have unprotected sex without birth control. Nothing would be more of a double dose of fun than an unplanned pregnancy, plus a maternity clothes shopping spree after you'd just gotten rid of her last maternity wardrobe.

So now we know that caring for a pregnant woman is more complicated than we first thought. Thanks to the pregnancy hormones, her mood and her needs are a moving target. These are the times where you can score some major points by helping take care of her and easing the difficulties of pregnancy in any ways possible. In addition to caring for her physically, don't forget to show her that you're loving the curves. Compliments and gentle, doctor-approved massages are a great way to do this.

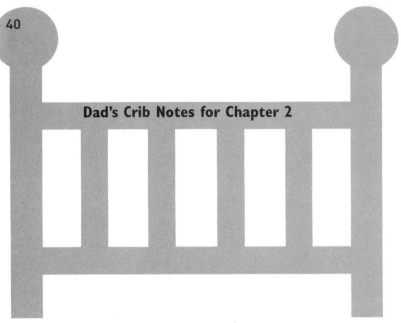

Dad's Crib Notes for Chapter 2

- She will need your help as she tackles changes caused by hormones, potentially including morning sickness.
- You may need to take on some extra cooking and cleaning duties—it's more manly than it sounds!
- You'll want to help her deal with her rapidly changing body. Hot tip: fat jokes are not the way to go.
- Pregnancy massage is best left to the experts, but there are some light, doctor-approved massage techniques you can master that she will greatly appreciate.
- As long as your doctor approves, pregnancy sex is all good.
- Exercise is good for the gander, and you too, goose. (Boring disclaimer: I mean doctor-approved exercise).
- It's getting time to suck it up and buy her some maternity clothes. Wearing your old T-shirts is not an acceptable fashion statement.

CHAPTER 3

Home Away from Home: The Doctor's Office

Once you've impregnated your BMP, you'll be given a fairly simple choice: attend the doctor's appointments or never have sex with her again. But you're not worried. You feel you're doing your job by staring at the pretty nurses and reading magazines. Be prepared: you will pay for this inactivity at a later date. To stave off being voted out of the relationship, bring a list of questions with you for the doctor. By the way, you're signed up for about sixteen of these things before the birth actually takes place!

> *By the way, you're signed up for about sixteen of these things before the birth actually takes place!*

Don't expect the doctor to give you all the information you need without being asked. Some of these offices have a revolving door so the doctor can come in, bless the proceedings, and keep moving to the next patient without breaking stride. So talk fast.

What Kind of Health Professional Does She Want?

Your BMP may already have a secret-lady-parts doctor (aka: gynecologist) whom she goes to. Many gynecologists are also obstetricians, so they can deliver babies for their patients. So unless you see a diploma from Bubba's Online Med School, then you shouldn't interfere with the relationship your partner has already established with her doctor.

Obstetrician/Gynecologist

Most pregnant women choose to have an obstetrician/gynecologist (OB/GYN) oversee prenatal care and delivery. If she has one of these already in her life, you're good to go. If you want to see an OB/GYN and don't have a go-to doctor filling this role, then you'll need to find a good one.

First and foremost, you'll want to find out what doctors accept your insurance coverage or are part of your health-care network. Between the checkups beforehand and the actual birth, the total financial cost of pregnancy can get too steep for you to even consider paying out of pocket.

Next, you must know that not every doctor has privileges at every hospital. So, if you have a preferred hospital—either because of reputation or location)—choosing a doctor with privileges there would be your next selection criteria.

It's also a good idea to ask questions about the doctor's opinion toward different procedures such as C-sections and induction. Some doctors will have a higher percentage of

C-section deliveries, which may show that the doctor executes this procedure as a first alternative, sometimes sooner than others might. The doctor's opinions on the matter should mirror your own as closely as possible, because if the meconium hits the fan in the delivery room, you'll most likely be following your doctor's orders. There just won't be time for a lot of discussion.

The selection process is also a good time to discuss any specific criteria your BMP might have. She may prefer a female doctor. Perhaps her friend had an especially good or bad experience at a certain hospital and she wants to take that into consideration. Other criteria may be the types of equipment the hospital has on hand, available reviews, and recommendations from friends, family, or coworkers.

Midwife

What does a midwife do? Is this term a code word for "transition wife," as when you no longer have a second wife but you know you're on your way to a third? Actually, a midwife is a specialist trained to deliver in low risk pregnancies. Some midwives—certified nurse-midwives—are trained and certified as nurses, and others—known as direct-entry midwives—learn through apprenticeships. Both types of midwives are frequently used in the case of a home birth. Sometimes they're associated with a physician, and sometimes not. Some doctors have deservedly gotten the reputation as impersonal directors for the birthing process. It may not be what you want, and midwives can offer an alternative. They are more about forming a partnership with you and your BMP. Besides, they do know natural ways to relieve your BMP's labor pain, so you may want to consider this option.

A midwife is a specialist
trained to deliver in low-risk pregnancies.

Doula

What's a doula? It's a question that's on the minds of men everywhere. Is it something sexual? Can I make money from this? Should we start a website?

Simply put, a doula is a pregnancy expert for hire, someone who helps support your partner while the doctor or midwife takes care of the medical details. Doulas serve as informed and experienced teammates during the birthing process. It's true, the angel on your shoulder is thinking that your BMP can use all the help available, even if it clouds the water on where you fit in. The devil on your other shoulder is whispering that maybe the doula can relief some of your pressure by providing added emotional support.

Instead of giving in to the angel or devil, think of a doula as an additional teammate. A really well-informed, experienced teammate who can help get your BMP safely through pregnancy. But not a teammate who can take your place on the team as the father and person who will be intimately involved in raising this baby.

Doulas can take the time to provide explanations and information the doctors won't or don't have time for. And they are often trained in the art of pregnancy massage, which naturally reduces pain during labor. But having a doula doesn't mean you get to sit in the recliner reading the paper while everything happens around you.

The Lowdown on Doctor's Office Visits

Pregnant women have lots and lots of appointments. Why so many? Because the doctor (or midwife) has to confirm that everything is progressing normally at key checkpoints along the way. You may think this fact doesn't have much to do with you until your BMP starts asking on what dates you can make yourself available. Then you'll realize that you're expected to be at most of, if not all of, the aforementioned doctor's appointments. In a perfect world, you would skip happily into each and every one, holding hands with your BMP all the while. But most of us live in the real world, which may lead to you having to ask yourself . . . .

Which Appointments Do I Attend?

You may not be able to attend every appointment. There are a lot of them, with more at the end of the pregnancy. From weeks 36 to 40, your partner is going every other week, and if, God forbid, you make it past that point, from week 40 on you'll have appointments every few days until the baby comes home to roost. You can also expect more appointments if your BMP or the baby have any complicating factors, such as gestational diabetes.

Take a few minutes to jot down a few questions you may have. It will reinforce that you're fully engaged in the pregnancy project, and perhaps even impress your woman. If your testosterone levels are dropping quickly enough, you can get your partner involved in coming up with some questions as a fun game the two of you play together. So, to that end, we'll look at which appointments are traditionally the most important.

Disclaimer: *Skip appointments at your own risk.*

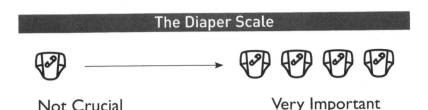

Not Crucial   Very Important

First Visit

Other than the actual birth, this is probably the most important appointment. You may be meeting the doctor for the first time yourself. You'll need to fill out all of the initial paperwork. Your partner will want you there for support. Many, many tests will be performed this day, including one to confirm the pregnancy, and this will be new and scary for both of you. Circle this one on your calendar in neon.

Importance:

Second Visit

This usually occurs about a month after the first visit. Some of the freshness and mystery is gone, as well as some of the apprehension. This visit is a little like blowing through the drive-through. The doctor checks your BMP's blood pressure, sugar levels, protein levels, weight, and sanity. Barring any abnormalities, the doc or midwife doesn't perform any new tests or discover any vital information, such as whether your child is destined to have abnormally large feet. Warning: Some doctors decide to listen to Junior's heartbeat for the first time at this appointment. Make sure you know if the doc plans to do this before you skip the appointment to go to Hooters with your coworkers.

Importance: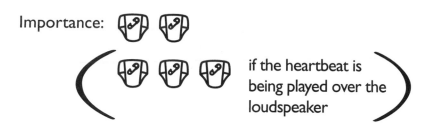

if the heartbeat is
being played over the
loudspeaker

Third Visit

Traditionally, this visit is a pretty big deal. As you reach the neighborhood of sixteen weeks, you're mathematically out of the scariest portion of the pregnancy, when a miscarriage is most likely to occur. The doctor fulfills her urine fetish again and checks your BMP's blood pressure and weight.

You'll be listening to the baby's heartbeat at each appointment pretty much from here on in. Your BMP's team of medical professionals will be measuring your BMP's fundal height, which actually doesn't involve mushrooms at all but simply measures the approximate size of your baby. The measurement is taken, usually in centimeters, from the top of the uterus to the top of the pelvic bone.

Importance:

Fourth Visit

The fourth visit is another eventful one. Urine, weight, heartbeat, fundal height, and blood pressure are taken. You should know the drill by now. But what makes this appointment noteworthy? This is usually the magical ultrasound appointment. Despite what your sorely lacking male brain tells you, this procedure is not done to identify the sex of the baby. Its true purpose is to check for all of the organs, fingers, and toes. You also get a picture of the baby, which is a major bonding experience, as we discussed in Chapter 1, in the "Get Into Bondage—No, Really" section.

Importance:

To Infinity . . . and Beyond!

The tests at each appointment become fairly similar from this point forward. The problem is, you can't always tell if these visits are trivial and eminently skippable, or if you really need to be there. If everything goes as planned, they will seem slightly repetitive to you, and you'll be wondering why you're missing work.

The key here is to remember that the alternative to these boring, repetitive visits would be a visit where something is wrong with the mother or child. This is obviously a worst-case scenario, so unlike a first date in which extreme boredom signals us that yet again we have underestimated the importance of personality versus looks, we will celebrate and embrace boredom when it comes to these doctor's visits.

Testing 1, 2, 3 . . .

So what exactly is going on with all these tests? Only Lance Armstrong will be more tested than your poor woman. Let's see exactly what the doctor is doing, starting with the first visit:

- **Complete medical history.** The doctor will want to know about any chronic illnesses, previous major illnesses, surgeries, drug allergies, what vitamins and supplements your BMP is on, and any medications she's taking. Both of your family medical histories will be reviewed for any genetic defects or chronic diseases. The doctor will be asking for information about any past miscarriages, abortions, and any other events along these lines. All of this is to help build a record and context to help your BMP and your child through any potential problems that may arise during the pregnancy.

- **Complete physical.** This involves all of the basics: height, weight, blood pressure, bra size. The doc will also be conducting a vaginal exam, and an examination of the pelvic areas. Blood pressure and weight will be checked at every visit.

- **Urine tests.** These measure excess sugar, protein, and white blood cells, which could indicate an illness. The urine is also checked for signs of unwanted bacteria and illegal drug use.

- **Blood tests.** These measure your BMP's antibodies and immunity to diseases such as rubella. One test also measures whether your woman has anemia and may need iron supplements.

- **Sexually transmitted disease tests.** These tests detect signs of syphilis, gonorrhea, hepatitis B, chlamydia, and HIV. If your partner has any of these, certain procedures and steps will be taken to help prevent them from harming the baby.

- **Genetic tests.** If genetic problems are indicated by medical history or ethnic background, the doctor may test for markers for cystic fibrosis, sickle-cell anemia, and a whole list of other genetic disorders.

- **And of course a Pap smear.** This will check for signs of cervical cancer.

Don't you feel well informed? These tests are the ones mainly performed at the first doctor's office visit. Let's see some of the other major tests:

- **Around weeks 15 to 18, the doctor will perform a "triple-screen" blood test,** which checks for possible birth defects. It's called a triple-screen test because three chemicals (with really long and complicated names that I'm not going to try to spell) are screened for. If they're there, it indicates that the baby may be at higher risk of having a problem such as Down syndrome or neural tube defects.
- **Glucose-tolerance test.** At about 28 weeks, blood is drawn (again) and diabetes testing is done.
- **At week 35 to 37, a Group B strep test is performed.** Blood is not drawn this time. No, this time the doc takes a vaginal and rectal swab. Somewhere between 20 to 40 percent of healthy women may have these bacteria present in the body. If they're there, you don't want the bacteria to be passed to the baby, so the doctor will take necessary precautions to make sure it isn't.
- **During the second trimester, ultrasounds are sometimes performed.** They may be done earlier in high-risk pregnancies or if the doc thinks there may be more than one baby in there. An ultrasound is like the scanner used at airports. But instead of looking for weapons or getting a perverse thrill as the more attractive passengers come through, the technician is

checking on your baby to make sure all of the vital parts are there.

Be sure to ask the doctor any questions you may have about any of the tests and what they're for. At the sight of all these tests, you may begin to wonder what exactly is going on. You can bet if you're feeling this way, your BMP might be doubly freaked out. It is *her* blood they're taking, after all. The fact that the staff is probably processing the tests without much personality or enthusiasm doesn't do much to put you at ease. This is where previewing what will happen during each doctor's office visit and researching the purpose of each procedure comes in handy. If you're properly prepared, you can put your BMP at ease about what's going on. Then guess who looks like a big smoothie?

Most obstetricians and midwives practice in groups, so even though she has "her" obstetrician, during her various appointments she'll see different doctors in the group.

Another note here about the doctors you and your BMP will be visiting: Most obstetricians and midwives practice in groups, so even though she has "her" obstetrician, during her various appointments she'll see different doctors in the group. This is done because whatever practitioner in the group happens to be on call at the time will be the one who delivers your brand-new child. The odds are in favor of the doctor or midwife you liked the least being the one who shows up that magical night. I wish you could gamble on these things; it would be easy money.

If your BMP's obstetrician or midwife doesn't practice in a group, he or she will still have a backup doctor that you and the mother of your child will want to meet before the delivery. You will want to make sure that there isn't anything in your birth plan that is a problem for that person. You also want to give the backup some of the screening that brought you to your primary doctor. Make sure her attitudes toward certain procedures match up with yours and that you feel you can trust her. Chances are, the backup doc has similar attitudes to the primary doc, but it doesn't hurt to ask a few questions.

If You're at Risk for Multiples

You mean I might end up with more than one of these things?

Yes, it can happen, especially if you're one of a growing number of people who use science to enhance your chances of getting pregnant. Using fertility drugs or the complicated process of IVF can lead to multiple babies at one time. Sometimes God just decides you're bored and gives you more than one to keep you busy. Either way, get ready for at least twice the fun!

To anyone who's having multiples, I can only advise a few things from my friends who have had this experience. First, when you get the news, stay positive, because she is scared too. Second, focus on the positive as much as possible, because having twins right off the bat is like taking doctoral-level courses in your first year of higher education. If you're having triplets, go ahead and try to adopt two more so you can get a reality show.

What Do I Do If Something Goes Wrong?

This pregnancy thang is all about having a plan. You'll plan three alternative routes to the hospital. You and your BMP will figure out a birth plan denoting what kind of drugs she'll take (if any), where the birth will take place, and who is allowed to be present. So it only makes sense that you would formulate a plan for problems, as painful and scary as it is to do so.

The thought of something happening to your unborn child sparks panic in anyone. If something were to happen, you might have trouble thinking straight. So it's best to prepare for this type of situation when you are calm, cool, and collected. Here is a list of recommended phone numbers to keep on hand. For redundancy, and in case your cell phone is dropped, run over, or swept out to sea, please keep a paper copy in your home, in her purse, and in your wallet.

1. In emergencies, dial 911; this is more of a reminder for when everyone freaks out and your brain locks up
2. Local emergency-room number
3. Your doctor's number or after-hours answering service
4. Insurance information
5. Your BMP's health information, including any allergies to medication
6. Family contact information

Along the pregnancy journey, there are many things that can crop up. Maybe there's a miscarriage, and both you and your partner will need to heal. Time is the only thing that will have a dramatic impact on how miserable you feel. But if having children is important to you both, try to find the courage to try again. I know we did. Maybe you find out your child has a birth defect or some other issue. Notice that the word "problem" is not used here. I have met parents of children with autism or another condition who have boundless love for their children. I am not going to say it doesn't require effort, or that there aren't difficult times, but in my experience the love is always strong. For these issues there is no platitude or foolproof advice I can give. Hold each other tight and talk to each other, no matter how tough it gets.

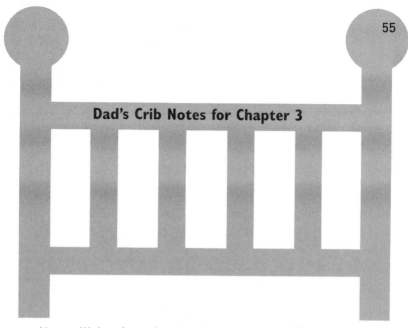

Dad's Crib Notes for Chapter 3

- You will begin going to the doctor's office on a regular basis. You're going to feel like you're there often enough to start paying rent. Don't miss any of the appointments if you can help it; some pretty cool stuff takes place along the way.
- While I referenced your doctor, you may select other health-care-provider options, such as a midwife or doula.
- Your BMP will be undergoing more tests than an Olympic athlete. These are mostly to ensure that your child is developing safely.
- As difficult as it is to think about, make sure you have a plan in place just in case any emergencies arise. Keep your insurance information and the names and numbers of your provider around at all times.

PART 2

The Second Trimester

The second trimester holds many joys in its ample bosom for you to enjoy. Its cups overflow with reasons to celebrate, like the halfway point of the pregnancy, some respite and stability for a time before the big event, and hopefully, a lessening of morning sickness.

For most of you, the worry of miscarriage will pass during this time. As for your BMP, get ready for some really visible changes. Although this is seen as the least-difficult trimester for many pregnant women, make sure you continue to offer support. Monthly doctor's visits will continue up until week 20, and then they'll pick up again to between every two to three weeks.

So this is a trimester to regroup and prepare yourself for the hectic third trimester that will be here before you know it.

CHAPTER 4

Ch-Ch-Ch-Changes . . .

As your BMP enters the second trimester, you begin to suspect she's smuggling something beneath her shirt. You figure either the baby is really beginning to show or your woman is a drug mule for a Mexican cartel.

This is the trimester where the most growth and change occurs. Some good news that should help you stay strong is that sometime soon your BMP's energy will be making a comeback (sort of like the 2004 Red Sox). Her trips to the restroom should start to decrease, so you'll no longer be tempted to suggest an adult diaper for her when the two of you go out in public together. Unfortunately, constipation can become more common now.

On the plus side, her breast tenderness should be decreasing, and speaking of breasts, they should also be getting larger. So you see, there's plenty of good news for both of you. Hey, tiger, it might even be time for you to get a closer look.

The most important thing a father
can do for his children is to love their mother.
—Theodore M. Hesburgh

Even More Change

As you enter Part Deux, your BMP will begin to show a baby bump and to gain weight. The gain will probably be more than the Freshman 15, because she did stuff herself with a baby, after all. But she will have that proverbial glow associated with pregnancy. That glow idea isn't just people being nice; the increased volume of blood during pregnancy often gives a pregnant woman's cheeks a rosy glow.

You may get to hear two words men least like to hear. "Not tonight" is number two on our list, with "vaginal discharge" taking the top spot. If you want more information about this, please do your own research. Just know that it's normal.

Here are some other common problems she'll be dealing with during the second trimester:

Heartburn

In this second frame, she could end up dealing with a cruel case of heartburn. Historically, it can be triggered by, well, eating. Traditional heartburn-inducing foods will probably be off the menu for a while.

Snoring

Lucky for you, you may have to deal with her snoring like a fat guy with allergies after a night of beer and wings. It's a grin-and-bear-it phenomenon. Although you get to hear the snoring, hear the complaining, and run to the store for cravings, the only thing worse would be actually having all of those things happening to you. Earplugs may do the trick, although I don't know how you hear the alarm to get up for work when your ears are full of earplugs.

I always thought sleeping in a different room didn't feel right. I mean, you signed up for the position of daddy and everything that goes with it. So hang in there and realize this is just the beginning of about two years of the sleep-deprivation program. One day you'll realize you officially qualify as a zombie, and the bandages for wrapping you from head to toe arrive on your doorstep in three to five business days.

Forgetfulness

Although recent research shows that "pregnancy brain" (aka "extreme memory loss brought on by growing a baby") doesn't exist, your BMP may have bouts of forgetfulness, whether it's because she's distracted by all that's going on or because of the magical pregnancy hormones. It can be harmless, like forgetting to turn off the lights or flush the toilet, but with luck she won't leave the car running when she gets home or leave the curling iron on and burn down the house. If these mental lapses get too bad, it may be time for you to leave for work after her, or hang a checklist by the door.

Insomnia

Around this time, your BMP could also begin to have trouble sleeping. Between having a human in her belly and the chemical imbalance the hormones cause, getting a good forty winks can be an issue. As with nonpregnant people, exercise can help your BMP sleep soundly. Late afternoon naps are not the best idea for her, and perhaps she should choose decaf for that after-dinner coffee. Caffeine or lengthy naps too close to her regular bedtime can cause her problems trying to get a sound night's sleep. Common sense will win the day.

That being said, weekend naps are probably a good idea to let her body catch up on any sleep deficit she has and let her body work on that very long to-do list that comes with pregnancy.

Mood Swings

Not only do the pregnancy hormones cause emotional swings you can't prepare for, but your BMP can't control or predict them. This puts you in a constant state of read-and-react. What sounds like a good idea at 11 A.M. may not sound like such a great idea at 11:15 A.M. We men need to stay ever vigilant, like Batman watching over Gotham City, in a state of constant readiness for our archrival, the evil and diabolical Hormone, to strike.

The Play-by-Play

As we've discussed ad nauseam, your BMP will be undergoing quite a few changes. For a good bit of the first trimester, most of those changes began to appear rather slowly. But things will begin to pick up. Let's take a look at some of the changes she will be undergoing, as well as a traditional time frame for them to occur:

Weeks 18–22

As your BMP's uterus (and thus her midsection) begins to stretch and expand, her body needs to change with it. She may get lower back pain, leg cramps, and tingling and numbness in her extremities. She may have bouts of dizziness, sleep problems, and swollen feet. The pregnancy hormones responsible for those mood swings can cause excess growth in her hair and nails, but if you nickname her Dragon Lady, keep it to yourself.

What about the baby? Oh yeah, forgot all about him. From weeks 18 through 21 several interesting things take place. In week 18 the ears' function generally comes online, allowing the baby to hear in the womb. In week 19, a protective, almost waxlike film covers your baby. As the baby's heart continues to grow, you can hear it beating, and it will generally pace about twice as fast as an adult's. By week 21, you can even hazard a guess about your baby's sleep patterns, as they become more regular. (Disclaimer: As with watching something on TV after a live football game or *American Idol*, all starting times are approximate.)

Discovering the Sex

Just as a heads-up, somewhere around weeks 20 to 22, your BMP will probably be getting her first ultrasound. Let's dispel a male urban legend right now: the sole purpose of this ultrasound is **not** to determine the sex of the baby. That's the impression many first-time fathers get. The purpose is actually to check on the baby, to make sure all the fingers and toes are there (not to mention organs).

When it comes to finding out the sex of your baby, it gets tricky. You can choose to find out or not; it's up to the two of you. Depending on what week the ultrasound takes place, that determination is from 95 to 99.9 percent accurate. Of course, the operator may not get a good view, and in today's world, we think anything less than 100 percent is 0 percent. You can usually depend on the technician's determination, though. It's up to you whether you want to only pick one name or paint the baby's room a gender-specific color.

Weeks 23–27

The area south of Belly Button Land and north of Privacy Boulevard is getting stretched, so aches and pains are the order of the day. As in previous weeks, her symptoms may include dizziness, heartburn, flatulence, leg cramps, and backaches. It's like having to suffer through the hangover without having had any of the fun.

Your BMP may also experience headaches and swelling in her ankles and feet. Her appetite should be hearty enough, so dump plenty of feed in the trough. Of course I'm joking! After these dainty meals, she could see some bleeding from her gums, especially when she brushes her teeth.

She should feel a definite uptick in the activity level and strength of motions from the baby. In fact, the baby will be kicking up a storm in there, and maybe even throwing some punches in for good measure. From all the angles and positions of the movements, many women start to wonder if they're carrying twins or if their child is destined to join a circus.

Weeks 28–31

In contrast to the fatigue she experienced in the first trimester, your BMP may now be feeling like she just chugged a couple of Red Bulls. But every woman's body is different, and even the same woman can have a different experience from one baby to the next.

More Than You Ever Wanted to Know about Mammary Glands

During this time, your BMP's mammary glands will start producing colostrum. For those of you who don't know: colostrum is a special substance, sometimes called "first milk," that contains antibodies to help keep Junior healthy. It's low in fat and high in carbs and protein, which may make it sound like a great pre-workout sports drink, but this is one fad that will never catch on. This fluid will nourish your baby if breastfeeding is on the agenda. A few days after birth, your BMP's mammary glands will start producing mature milk, which doesn't have colostrum in it, but which will still do a good job of helping Junior thrive.

If your BMP's breasts seem to have sprung a slight leak, don't be concerned. (Bonus: If she catches you sneaking a peek at her chest, for once you have a built-in excuse.) If her breasts and nipples look flat, she should consult the doctor or midwife. This is especially important if she plans to breastfeed.

Remind her to take any prenatal vitamins that have been prescribed and to drink lots of water for her overall health and a healthy pregnancy.

Exercise is still important too. It will get harder, because her balance is thrown off by the baby inside her . . . and also because smaller objects begin to orbit around her due to her size and gravitational pull. As she moves closer to the due date, her hips may widen slightly in preparation for the birth. In **no way** are you to notice this; the future of your relationship may hang in the balance.

Preeclampsia, or high blood pressure brought on by pregnancy, sometimes occurs in the second trimester. If your BMP experiences any of the common symptoms, including severe headaches, swelling in the face, nausea, or visual spots, she needs to contact the doctor immediately.

Preeclampsia, or high blood pressure brought on by pregnancy, sometimes occurs in the second trimester. If your BMP experiences any of the common symptoms, including severe headaches, swelling in the face, nausea, or visual spots, she needs to contact the doctor immediately.

Dealing with Braxton-Hicks

Braxton-Hicks contractions, also known as false labor pains, may be coming on. You can tell the difference between Braxton-Hicks and real contractions by a few differences:

1. **Timing.** Braxton-Hicks contractions don't follow a regular pattern, unlike real labor contractions.
2. **Pain.** Braxton-Hicks contractions do not generally bring pain. Real contractions, on the other hand . . . .
3. **Reaction to moving.** Movement, such as walking, often stops Braxton-Hicks contractions.

Of course, you do risk ending up on the television show *I Didn't Know I Was Pregnant* if you ignore every symptom that occurs, so take note. You can even help your BMP keep a journal of symptoms.

What Your Baby Is Doing

As the second trimester moves forward, your baby keeps growing. Baby will change from the size of your blue balls to larger than the size of a softball.

Your little angel will also begin to protest her entrapment by kicking your BMP. Said angel will also have some slight movement of fingers and toes. And, to the relief of all, Baby starts to look less alien, as eyes move to their appropriate spot.

For your unborn child during the second trimester, hair is where it's at. It's like a '60s revival in there! Research tells us that at this point your child looks like Cousin It. Or put another way, your baby is getting pretty hairy from head to toe. But it isn't time for an inutero laser hair procedure. The hair keeps Baby warm, and the unwanted fur will be gone in time for the first shot from your digital camera/phone/mp3 player. But if you have extreme hair issues on both sides of the family, maybe it's time for both a college savings plan and a laser hair-removal fund, at least for the shoulders and upper back.

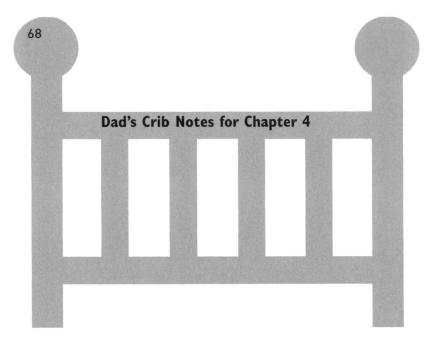

Dad's Crib Notes for Chapter 4

- You will start to notice many changes in your BMP, both physical and otherwise. Did someone shrink all of her shirts?
- When you have your first ultrasound, you'll have the opportunity to discover the sex of your child. Do you want to know if it's going to be a boy or a girl?
- She may experience Braxton Hicks, or false labor, contractions. It is advisable to know the differences between these and the real thing.

CHAPTER 5

Baby Stuff

This is going to be a piece of cake. How much stuff can a kid need? A few bottles, a few diapers, a crib? That's about it, right?

The simple answer is no. You're about to enter a previously unknown (to you) and bizarre universe with so many options available that you need to do a dizzying amount of research.

If you're planning to bottle-feed, your baby needs bottles, but what type of nipple are you going to use? Latex, silicon, and rubber are the most popular options, but which one is the best? I ask this in jest, as no man without children knows the answer to this question. But this example should at least give you a clue as to what you're up against. Where you seek simplicity, none actually exists. There are five different bottle warmers, and we like the Brand X crib, but they have a history of safety issues, so should we pick something different?

Are you beginning to see the light? Tackling all the possibilities for each product is a tough task for anyone. Just make sure you think about putting some honest effort into being informed on some of the more important items. Many websites are dedicated to the topic of buying baby stuff, along with moms' comments attached—kind of like your fantasy message board, but more serious, and actually providing useful information.

Many websites are dedicated to the topic of buying baby stuff, along with moms' comments attached—kind of like your fantasy message board, but more serious, and actually providing useful information.

Nesting

Aaaahhh. The joys of nesting. But what exactly is nesting? Nesting is the pregnant female's need to scrub, scrub, and then scrub some more until the entire house is germ-free in preparation for baby's arrival. Kitchen disposals will be deconstructed and scrubbed. You favorite pair of boxers from college may "accidentally" be thrown away. Your woman will feel the almost insatiable need to clean every nook and cranny of the kitchen, garage, attic, and refrigerator. No cleaning project will be left undone.

And you thought you were going to get to relax this weekend! In nature, males go out to hunt during this time. For us modern human males, the local bodega or grocery store just isn't far enough away for us to justify our "hunting" there to last all weekend and missing out on this pregnancy ritual.

Be ready for the honey-do list to grow to lengths unseen before now. Just know that, statistically, your man-cave is finished. On its last legs. The weakest of the herd. That man cave—where you used to watch football games and brag to your friends about how you *could* smoke cigars, but you just didn't want to—is about to be turned into a baby palace full of duckies, bunnies, and bright pastels. You had a good run, but now it's over. So get ready to go to the home-improvement store and pledge your love for light yellow or gender-neutral green. Get ready to buy all the most expensive everything (because you love your new baby-to-be, don't you)?

When preparing Baby's room, there are a few things you might want to remember:

1. Read reviews on cribs and check the manufacturers' past products for safety, especially if you're buying a "lightly used" crib. The U.S. Consumer Product Safety Commission keeps a list of recalled baby and children's items here: *www.cpsc.gov/cpscpub/prerel/ category/child.html*. Recalled toys are listed separately here: *www.cpsc.gov/cpscpub/prerel/category/toy.html*.

2. If you decide to paint Baby's room, remember that paint fumes are not the best for your BMP and the baby, so make sure you keep the area well ventilated. Waving the "free-beer" sign may be enough to convince friends to help.

3. Although ultrasound technicians are pretty good at determining the baby's sex, it doesn't hurt to purchase a few neutral-colored items.

4. "Specialty" baby stores charge double.

Don't go overboard. You can score some free baby items with a well-planned strategy for your baby shower.

The Baby Shower

I recently attended a friend's baby shower. I was yet again confused by the fact that no shower was offered and no babies were present. As I glanced around the room, I spotted ample food and drink, so I proceeded into the heart of the misnamed event. It was a couples' shower, which is basically a lame attempt to include the father in the pregnancy experience. Even though there was a football game on, it quickly became apparent that the only part of this gathering that the father-to-be could savor was the perfectly cooked steaks and the well-stocked bar. Everything else, from the decorations and ridiculous party games to the gifts themselves, was intended for the pregnant lady and her birth-canal-storming offspring to enjoy.

Meanwhile, my buddy sat idly by, not knowing what half the gifts were or how to use them. But I felt like he was looking at this event in the wrong way. With a little planning, a baby shower isn't an assault on your manliness—it's a way you can get your friends to help you stock the baby's room.

With a little planning, a baby shower isn't an assault on your manliness—it's a way you can get your friends to help you stock the baby's room.

Most men initially see the baby shower as a big ordeal they'd prefer to avoid. If that's how you feel, get over it, because it's probably going to happen. We know that at this point in your evolution as a man, the baby shower ranks below several other events you can think of, mostly involving professional sports, scantily clad women, great food, or, ideally, all three. You can guess how this thing is going down. Some super-enthusiastic "friend" will insist on it. You may want to make sure said friend is a real go-getter, and that she understands any budgetary restraints you're under.

Make sure the helpful friend is cool. If she isn't, maybe suggest that someone you trust "really had her heart set on doing our baby shower." This person will kill you for volunteering them, but at least you will have an ally on the inside. Babies make some people do crazy things. Your seemingly normal friend may turn into an overly enthusiastic psycho who will host a themed baby shower such as "Eco-Friendly Baby" (pre-order the Prius).

If you're not careful, you'll find yourself wrapped up in baby shower games, such as Guess Mom's Tummy Size and What Flavor of Baby Food Is This? These disasters can get out of hand in a hurry, so don't just zone out, or the next thing you know, your BMP will come up to you during the shower and tell you it's time for you to put on the diaper and baby hat like you agreed. That's what you get for mindlessly nodding yes when she talks to you during the game.

If your woman gives you a pass on the shower to go hang out with your buddies, buy her something nice. She's a keeper.

Registering

Make no mistake, there's nothing at this shower for you. You'll have to be on good behavior, and if you're lucky, you'll get to have the big game on in the background. The silver lining is that you don't have to pay for all this. In fact, this is an opportunity to get family and your buddies to pay for a bunch of stuff you'll have to buy anyway. When registering, think like Machiavelli. You want to register for things that cost $50 and up. No bottles, no socks, nothing under $10. You can pay for that stuff yourself. Be ready with the "I don't want other people dressing our child" excuse when your BMP wonders why you're so hot on registering for that bouncy seat.

When registering, just know that every new mommy will need a diaper bag. It's like a really big purse, with pockets for diaper-changing supplies instead of auxiliary makeup. Be ready for the wall of diaper bags. Every baby store has an entire wall dedicated to diaper bags with varying features. She'll want to look at all of them. It may take upwards of two hours. You may begin to feel lightheaded and see dancing babies in the aisles. Don't be frustrated when she ends up with the solid black one, possibly the first one she looked at. "I think you made a smart choice, you'll be a great mother" always earns brownie points.

Off-List Gifts

Once this shower is underway, be ready for the few guests who buy off-list. Apparently they found nothing suitable on your registry, thought everything was too expensive (you planned it this way), or decided they were just a little bit wiser about what you and your unborn child will need (which is especially funny if they don't have children).

Most likely, they waited until the last second and all of the best—or less expensive—items were gone, or the husband was feeling rebellious. Either way, don't you dare sweat it. You'll end up with a pretty good haul of gifts when the dust settles after the event. If gift opening begins to bore, just imagine having to buy all of this stuff yourself. That should help perk you up.

Step carefully and avoid stepping on any toes if a gift is something that you know right away won't be used in your house. If Auntie Ethel gives you an old handcrafted oak crib, try not to blurt out "Firewood!" as you toss it aside because you just read an article labeling these types of cribs unsafe. She isn't trying to hurt anyone, and when you see a gift horse, it's not kind to look them in the mouth, much less kick their teeth in. No, whether the gift costs $250 or is something you know will not be used, give the same amount of thanks and move on. If Ethel comes for a visit and notices her crib is not in use, then politely inform her about the information you discovered, and let's hope she understands.

Some Assembly Required

Now we arrive at a less desirable destination. You've tried your best to research some important items for your new child. Once you achieved product enlightenment, you shrewdly registered for those items you really, really, did not want to shell out big bucks for, not from your own wallet. You withstood the baby shower itself. You may even have suffered through the tasting of various flavors of mush from tiny jars while wearing a diaper and a bib. What could possibly be worse?

The answer appears in the small print of commercials where the manufacturer lets you know, in the vaguest terms possible, that "some assembly is required." What this really means is that the manufacturer hopes you can read advanced schematic drawings, are as bendable as an Olympic gymnast, and are extremely handy with an Allen wrench.

The best idea with a mountain of gifts in front of you needing assembly is to make sure all of them get done well in advance of Baby's arrival.

The best idea with a mountain of gifts in front of you needing assembly is to make sure all of them get done well in advance of Baby's arrival. Once the baby makes an appearance, the premium you'll place on sleep will make assembling these gifts difficult, to the point you'll be mentally cursing the people who gave them to you. So whether you want to assemble two per week or pull an all-night assembly party, just make sure the deed gets done in time.

Oh, and about the car seat: a sampling of 619 car seat installs in Pennsylvania in 2008 showed that almost 80 percent of them were installed incorrectly or were not the proper size for the child sitting in them. This isn't something you want to get wrong. Babies have limited strength, especially when considering the strength of their neck muscles versus the weight of their head, so make sure you get this right. Search the web for an event in your area on proper installation.

Choosing a Name

Stuff isn't all your kid needs. He or she also needs a name. This can be problematic. I say that only because if you screw this up, your child is doomed for life. It never seems fair that the parents who bestow curses upon their children in the form of horrific names should get to roam the Earth penalty-free. If your last name sets you up for obvious naming infractions, you, as a caring parent, need to take the situation out of play and not tempt fate. Mr. and Mrs. McCrackin have no business naming their son Phillip. And why would a nice churchgoing couple like the Pitts name their son Harry? C'mon, people, don't do these things to your kids.

The Name Game

No, I'm not talking about your internal debate on whether you're going to require your child to refer to you as "P-Diddy" or "Big Papi." I'm speaking of coming up with that perfect name for your child. Naming your child is a process that seems like it might be fun. In reality, it can be a trap-filled power struggle that you may not survive.

It starts with an innocent question like, "What names do you like?" This is the time to open the vault and break out your favorite name for a boy and a girl. You know, those names you think are really cool, that you've picked out over time but simply never told anyone about. After unveiling your favorite names for a boy or a girl, you sit back with a satisfied smile on your face, waiting for your BMP's look of admiration at your naming brilliance. Sadly, the girls' names you like will be met with under-the-breath comments such as, "Sounds like a stripper name." And the boys' names will get vetoed for reasons you never saw coming, such as, "It doesn't have the right number of syllables."

Baby-naming books only add to the confusion. After reading 500 or so names, you start talking yourself into names that really aren't that great. I just found a website pushing the name Bridger really hard for a baby boy. On the off chance that it's 2 A.M. and you've been at it for hours, you may actually fall prey to some baby-naming book's seductive argument for Bridger. When your BMP shoots it down, a fight ensues. So just be careful with overuse of naming resources and today's anything-goes mentality. It's a thin line between a cool new name and one that makes your kid the butt of many jokes.

A word of caution: never defend a name to the death just to assert your manhood. Your wife may eventually decide that if you feel that strongly about something involving your child, you should get your way, and you'll have a son named Ellison because you watched the University of Louisville's Never Nervous Pervis on ESPN Classic and decided to dig in your heels.

Dealing with Family Expectations

Beware the input of the family. Although they have fond memories of Aunt Beatrice and want your baby to carry the torch, you'll take the fall when your daughter sets the record for most high-school dances attended without a date. Tell family members who want a say to write their suggestions down on paper and deposit them into a box. After your family has gone home and it's just you and your BMP, break out a bottle of sparkling grape juice,* mock them endlessly, and then deposit the box in the trash can or burn it.

---

*If you thought I was going to say "bottle of wine," then you forgot that your BMP cannot drink. Please go back to the beginning of the book and start over.

You'll be just fine with your version of "Thanks for your thoughts and input on naming our child. Your opinion is important to us." The coast is now clear and you are free to return to playing the "I am NOT suggesting Charles just because I love Chuck Norris" game with your partner. Although *POW I, II*, and *III* were a pretty bad-ass movies.

A Naming Rule

Do not try to sneak in a name that represents something funny to you but if your wife finds out, you're dead. I know it's tempting. You're thinking that every time you see your child, you'll get a little giggle. Names of old girlfriends, that stripper you thought you loved in college, and your online avatar are off-limits. I hate to be the one to drop a heavy load on you, but your child will grow up and you'll end up feeling like a jerk.

Naming your child after a relative always sounds cool. But if you break out the family tree and find it full of Gertrudes and Harolds, then you have to give it up. Don't try to get fancy with "We'll call her Gert!" Her name has still preselected her to arrive solo at homecoming wearing Coke-bottle glasses. And don't think you can solve that problem with the use-the-middle-name-as-the-first-name strategy. That just confuses everyone, including the kid, who won't know what his monogram should really look like. Even if you aspire to be famous or simply rich, avoid the temptation to employ the celeb strategy of choosing confounding names. Apple doesn't sound cool as a person's name, even if your mother is Gwyneth Paltrow.

Now let's look at some specific naming recommendations. Eligible persons worthy of naming your children after can include great musicians and artists. Some say politicians (but my objection is that there aren't any great politicians). It's preferable to wait until these potential name givers are deceased—or at least really, really, old. This is mainly because prominent people can do some really stupid things. Imagine if in the early 1990s, as a hardcore Democrat, you decided to name your bouncing baby boy after President Bill Clinton. He would be slightly limited in his dating options, as he could never date from the pool of women named Monica. I am quite conflicted about the more recent trend of naming Junior after a city, state, or territory. I am for Dakota Fanning and Brooklyn Decker. Thumbs up. I think I would be willing to explore naming my unborn son Rome. But I'm not sure about Montana, because it carries too much baggage.

The lists of top ten names by year are a ripe orchard of naming ideas. Let's look at a sampling of the top ten from 2009 for boys and girls.

Girls

1. **Isabella.** It's a lot of name for a little girl in my opinion. Shouldn't Isabella be walking along the banks of the Seine? Perhaps on her way to eat escargots at a political rally for French workers to get more than their exploitive three months of vacation?
2. **Emma.** This reminds me of a plucky young teen with a can-do attitude. Perhaps I am just falling prey to the Emma Roberts hype machine.

3. **Sophia.** Again, this one seems a bit outsized for a cute little girl. Who can really follow in Sophia Loren's footsteps? There's nothing like putting on the pressure by forcing comparisons with Sophia Loren, who was once quoted as saying, "You have to be born a sex symbol. You don't become one. If you're born with it, you'll have it even when you're 100 years old."

4. **Abigail.** I find this one kind of clunky, but it's still pretty in the long run. Please do not shorten this to Gail. It's a tough name to do really well with unless you are ridiculously pretty, personable, and humorous. Plus, if you read the name Abigail slowly enough, it turns into "A big Gail." I think we all agree you can do better elsewhere.

5. **Mia.** If after much consideration you decide to name your daughter Mia, she'll hopefully turn out to be more Mia Hamm (Gold-winning soccer player) than Mia Wallace (heroin-snorting Pulp vixen).

Boys

1. **Alexander.** Make his middle name The Great. How cool would that be? Alexander The Great Pfeiffer. This child is going places.

2. **Joshua.** If it's good enough for U2 and their tree, then it's fine with me.

3. **Daniel.** It's a little too Karate Kid for me. Just make sure you make him paint the fence, sand the deck, and wax the car. Then at least he can kick the local bully's ass and get the girl.

4. **Noah.** It is hard to go wrong with a Biblical name. It's classic, and God-approved. When he reaches for an umbrella and packs your two Weimaraners into the car, make sure you stay close to him and get on the boat.

5. **Anthony.** Lots of famous people and characters to think about here. He could be Head of the Family someday. Of course, I mean starting his own family, not the stereotypical families in *The Sopranos* or *Goodfellas*.

Names to Avoid

While we're visiting this area, let's cover some names to avoid. I would skip this section, but every year I meet more and more people who can't seem to get away from these awful names. Once ink dries on the birth certificate, then all of my sarcasm just seems mean. We know naming is subjective, but please consider that you may be dooming your child to a life of beatdowns and no lunch money.

1. **Stanley.** This sounds like your child will be a vacuum cleaner salesman, or a sad sack bald guy in a tweed coat. There is one and only one loophole here: if he becomes a hockey player, he can probably survive.

2. **Jezebel.** No less authority than the Bible has deemed that your little girl will become a harlot. Do you really want to lay this label on her just after she exits the womb?

3. **Oprah.** I don't know if this one ever really picked up a lot of steam, but let's face facts. We think of an affable woman with weight problems.
4. **Henrietta.** See Hippo, Hungry Hungry.
5. **Bertha.** Just bad. Golf-club maker Callaway callously named its largest club the Big Bertha. There weren't even enough Bertha supporters around for a decent class-action lawsuit.

My Challenge to You

A $100 reward goes to the guy who convinces his BMP to choose the middle name Danger. Don't worry about your son; he'll have females all over him, and men will admire him. "Danger is my middle name." That and a driver's license backing up this claim would have to be the easiest pickup line you could ever create. In a way, you would be removing one of the hardest and most intimidating experiences from your son's life. That is unless he turns out to be 5'5" and 120 pounds. Then I sure do hope he can write killer poetry or become a movie star.

What to Call the Grandparents

While we're on the subject of names, just remember that the grandparents will be getting new names also. Most grandparents go by the traditional Grandma and Grandpa. Some grandparents who are younger—or simply young at heart— might not enjoy the over-the-hill moniker of Grandpa. It's always fun to stick it to my dad by dropping a casual Pops or Gramps his way. It keeps him honest.

It can also be tricky with step-grandparents. First names are good, or you can just ask them what they'd like to be called. Or let your child dictate—grandchildren can usually do no wrong in their grandparents' aging, far-sighted eyes.

Babies, of course, will go with the flow, so if you present this gray-haired adult as Maw, the child won't know any better. I have also seen a child mispronounce a grandparent's name, and it ended up sticking.

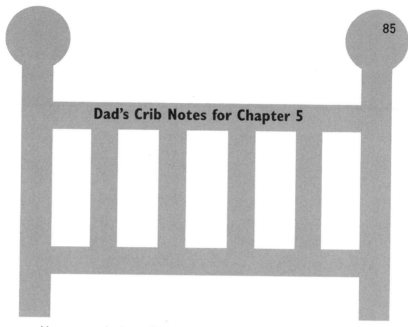

Dad's Crib Notes for Chapter 5

- Your new baby will need many items, including a crib, clothing, and bottles. Do some research on these before purchasing. Some brands have a higher occurrence of safety problems or recalls; stay away from those particular brands.
- You may notice your BMP showing some signs of nesting, or preparing the home for the impending arrival of your baby. She may also want your help and input tackling these projects!
- Get ready to attend the possible upcoming baby shower. Registering for gifts can be an adventure.
- The good news? Your shower guests will come bearing gifts. The bad news: there may be "some assembly required" (for you).
- If you haven't already, you'll need to complete the surprisingly difficult task of agreeing on a name for your baby.
- Depending on your family situation, the grandparents may need new names as well.

CHAPTER 6

Getting Ready
for the Delivery

We are reaching a critical time. If there's anything we've discussed in previous chapters that you've been waiting to do, it's time to get in gear. Because now we are getting into the most important parts of the preparation for your child's arrival: the learning process about the hospital, the different delivery scenarios, and having a birth plan in mind.

Hospital Logistics

When it comes time for the baby to be delivered, the most important thing to remember is how to find the hospital. You don't know from where you'll be traveling, what time of day it may be, or how quickly you'll need to get there. A baby is truly on his own schedule. So you could be screeching into the emergency admissions area, delivery assured to take place at any moment, or, if delivery involves the words "induction" or "C-section," you could be arriving at a more

measured pace. But it behooves you to be prepared for any
and all situations. Here is what you'll need to know.

Fastest Route

Her water breaks in the middle of the night. You sleep-
ily inform her you need just ten more minutes of sleep. She
kicks you. You should have the absolute best route to the
hospital or birth center mapped out cold in your mind. You
should be able to navigate it backwards and forwards with
no problem.

Alternate Route

Traffic, construction, accident, funeral procession? No
problem. You're taking the lead. Over the hills and through
the woods you go, and voilà! You arrive at the hospital safe
and sound.

Drop-off Area

Once you arrive, pull out your walkie-talkie and
announce to your advance team, "The eagle has landed." But
where do you drop off your guest of honor? You don't want
to be squinting at signs on a dark and rainy night while the
baby is crowning. You need to know exactly where to go.

Alternate Alternate Route

If you live in a city where lots and lots of driving is the
norm, plan ahead for this possibility as well. Maybe you're
at the shopping mall on the other side of town when the
blessed event begins. Or at Grandma's, way out in the country. Get your routes from all likely locations straightened
out ahead of time, and keep copies on her person and in all
the vehicles. Who know? Maybe she'll be shopping with a

friend who will need your directions. GPS is pretty good, but do you want to be as prepared as possible or not?

Getting Your BS Degree (Baby Safety, of Course)

As the saying goes, you can prepare for the worst and hope for the best. So, as for planning for the worst, here are some of the steps you should consider:

- **Infant CPR class.** It's not a cheery thought, I know, of being in a situation where your child needs CPR. But that high school health-class training was a long time ago, and you were staring at the head cheerleader while she practiced CPR and you wished you were the mannequin. So take a few hours and get to class. If you bring it up first, it will score you some brownie points with your BMP for being so smart.
- **Infant first-aid kits.** Purchase a kit for the home, and one for each and every car Junior may be riding in.
- **Sleep planning.** SIDS—Sudden Infant Death Syndrome—is the leading cause of death among children one month to one year old. One of the most frightening facts about SIDS is that doctors aren't exactly sure what causes it. One thing they do know is that sleeping on the stomach is one of the leading factors in these deaths. Thus, sleep planning. You'll want to put baby to sleep on her back. In addition, remove all stuffed animals, blankets, pillows, and the like from the crib. Baby can get tangled up in them, choke, or have trouble breathing. You should also alternate

the position of the baby's head from night to night, to keep Junior from developing a flat spot and getting ridiculed by the other babies in baby gymnastics class.

Birthing Class

Birthing class is an event no man can ever be properly prepared for. The descriptions from your buddies do not do justice to the mental scarring you will suffer. It all seems innocent enough. You pack a lunch, hold hands on your way out the door, and exchange smiles with the other happy couples as you arrive. You're feeling the flow, and you don't even protest wearing the nametag the happily medicated instructor asks you to wear. You try to block comments about the other attendees out of your head, like, "If she wasn't pregnant, she'd be really hot." They are inappropriate and you are feeling the happy-happy joy-joy of impending fatherhood.

The class starts innocently enough, with introductions and a few segments relating to the responsibilities of being a parent. There may be a couple there who already has children and simply showed up for a refresher. Be careful with them, as they're simply here to prove how smart they are about parenting.

Just as their know-it-all act is wearing on you, the class moves on to a time-honored tradition. The VCR comes out and they slap in the porno-like birthing film from the 1970s, with the funkified music and body parts in all of their glory. Were those humans? Good Lord. Who knew pubic hair could grow that long? You won't be able to banish from your brain the images from this film, and it will come into your mind uninvited over and over again. The vision on this VHS tape will be seared into your brain forever. Those things should come with some sort of warning: "May be hazardous to your sex life," or maybe, "May cause permanent blindness."

My advice is to be prepared and close your eyes when the main event comes on. It's not like you learn anything, and your sweet bride, who, during the delivery will probably be floating on painkillers, won't look anything like that monster you just saw. Benefits also include the fact that you won't have to fight nausea throughout the rest of the class.

After the class, you will return to your life. You and your BMP will have grown closer and have another bonding experience under your belts. She doesn't seem affected by anything she saw or heard in there, which makes you wonder if she did some black-ops work for the CIA in Iraq. You, on the other hand, are changed forever, and are ready and willing to make considerable sacrifices if somebody would just remove the images you just witnessed from your brain.

Hospital Tour

At first, determining the layout and available amenities that are offered at the local hospital probably doesn't hold much allure for the average man, or even for the below-average man, for that matter. Hospital planners tend to focus on caring for patients, profitability, and elimination of lawsuits. The need for their guests or visitors to be entertained during their stay is secondary, if it's even considered at all. But to a man who has impregnated a woman he loves, a change in perspective is needed. This is where his new child is going to be brought into the world, and where he will be spending a couple of uncomfortable, sleepless nights. So get to know this place like the back of your hand.

How to start? Try the hospital tour. That clean and fresh hospital smell hits you . . . ahhhhh. Take it all in. This is the place where your life will be changed forever. Unlike with marriage, there's no party sending you off into parenthood. Just you and your chosen one facing down one of the most exhilarating and terrifying experiences known to man. It cannot be overstated the degree of difficulty of what lies ahead.

Intimidated yet? Surely I'm overdoing it? You may be asking yourself, "What should I do now?" Well, the good news is that you're doing what you should be doing right now. Touring and researching the hospital where your child will enter the world is the first step. As you tour, take note of the layout. More and more of these facilities are moving toward the "living room" approach. There is the main bed for Mom. Yes, that small couch in the corner of the room is where you'll be sleeping for several days. There's also a TV, and usually a DVD player and a CD player. If not, you may be allowed to bring these items with you. Some facilities provide a rocking chair for you or Mom to hold Baby in.

Make special note of the nursery area. Although your first reaction may be that you would never send your newborn to be watched by strangers, experienced parents know better. Newborns are not born ready to be on our schedule, and may be up through some or most of the night. So send

Junior to be watched by the professionals. It may be the last gasp of sleep you get for some time.

Birth Plan

What birth plan? You wait until the baby's ready, you go to the hospital, she spits it out, and you're good to go, right?

No, genius, plans need to be made. Putting some clothes for her, you, and the baby in a travel bag by the front door doesn't cut it, either.

Here are some of the exciting and controversial decisions you'll have the fun of making. Remember, you don't really get input, but you do serve as a listening post for *every* conceivable scenario. She'll decide whether the delivery will be vaginal or cesarean; in pain or drugged; in stirrups and handcuffs or with free movement, walk, stretch, or jump rope; with freedom to feast or ice chips; breastfeeding or bottle; circumcised or foreskin; and with an episiotomy or not. (When you learn what that last one means, you'll start to believe maybe Eve did screw up in the Garden of Eden and God did punish accordingly.) Do you feel the responsibility of adulthood crushing your spontaneity?

In addition to these basics, you'll need to have answers prepared ahead of time for a few other questions. Besides your health-care provider, who are you going to call? Do you want your parents there? In-laws? Brothers? Sisters? If the extended family includes younger children, are they coming to see the baby show? Who are you sending out to get you some real food? Are you bringing a CD player for atmosphere and to build to a crescendo of the Beatles' "Come Together"? You'll also want to take things you liked from all of the classes and research you've done and put them into play. You did read those books and pay attention in class, right?

Cord Blood

While umbilical cord blood won't be collected until the actual birth, you need to decide about it beforehand. Medically, we now have the capability to use a baby's cord blood in the treatment of many conditions, such as various cancers, genetic diseases, blood disorders, and immune-system problems. There is research underway to use cord blood in treating cases of diabetes and cerebral palsy. So, the question is do you want the blood from the baby's umbilical cord to be taken out and stored for potential medical use? Twenty years ago, it wasn't really a viable option, but it's a growing trend today.

Once you've decided on a birth plan, take that plan (aka, "book of wishes") and schedule time to go through it with your doctor or midwife. She may add some information you didn't think of or tell you whether any portions of your plan are a tad, um, unrealistic. But an in-depth discussion with a qualified and informed individual will help you refine your plan. Who knows? Maybe you nailed it and this talk will only serve to strengthen how you're already feeling. Either way, modification or validation, it's worth everyone's time to do it.

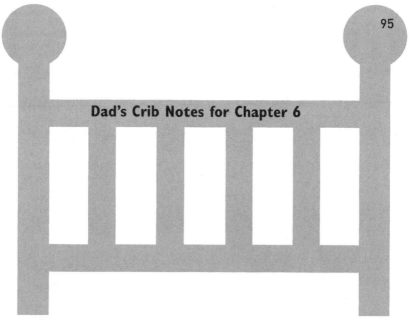

Dad's Crib Notes for Chapter 6

- Get to know the best routes to the hospital you've chosen for your child's birth. You never know where you might be when labor starts.
- Parents-to-be should strongly consider receiving infant medical training and purchasing infant first-aid kits for their home and vehicles.
- Attending birthing class and taking a tour of your hospital are great ways for parents to prepare themselves for the big day.
- Your birth plan will help you research and make important decisions about the birth of your child beforehand. When critical decision points come up during the pregnancy, you'll be ready.
- There is a growing trend to preserve newborns' umbilical cord blood. Talk to a qualified health-care provider if this is something you're considering.

PART 3

Third Trimester

If you've made it this far, congratulations! Although, in reality, your BMP is doing most of the heavy lifting (no jokes, please). Now is the time to line up paternity leave, make sure those names are the right ones, and double-check the birth plan.

Although it doesn't seem possible, doctor's appointments will become even more frequent toward the end of the trimester. From week 32 forward, your woman may gain a pound a week. As the doctor will remind you, it's important for your BMP to stay hydrated and stay diligent with her vitamins.

You are now on a collision course with delivery. Toward the end of the pregnancy, your exhausted partner will be hoping for the birth, and the sweet relief that follows, to mercifully come.

CHAPTER 7

Things to Squeeze In Before the Baby Squeezes Out

There is a growing trend today where the children are not only the focus of the family, but are the sole focus of the family. Parents cut back or cut out hobbies and social activities, and even spend the majority of the disposable income on the children. So while you shouldn't get an iPad for yourself and tell your kids there will be no Christmas this year, the best way to maintain sanity is the lost art of balance.

"What is this 'balance' you speak of?" you might be muttering to yourself. It is the art form of giving attention to the important things in life and keeping yourself sane. This is a good chance to practice keeping a balance. Up until now it has been all about Junior, and he hasn't even arrived yet. So make some time for yourselves.

Taking a Vacation

You may want to squeeze in one last vacation during this last stanza of the pregnancy. As long as you get a permission slip signed by your doctor, you should be good to go. I'm assuming you're with me here when I say the idea is for you to go with your BMP. So don't be totally obtuse when it comes to selecting a destination. Mardi Gras, Vegas, and a tour of wine country = not the best destinations.

Of course, it may not be the pace you've been used to on past vacations. Keeping a flexible, lighter-than-usual schedule will help you handle whatever's going on with her ever-changing body. It's a change for both of you, and a precursor to the not-being-able-to-get-away-on-a-moment's-notice type of lifestyle that's headed your way. Depending on how far out you're planning, you may want to buy the much-maligned travel insurance. Then if she gets so sick you can't go, you won't be fuming over the lost funds.

Depending on how far out you're planning, you may want to buy the much-maligned travel insurance. Then if she gets so sick you can't go, you won't be fuming over the lost funds.

As for eating on the road, try to have some sort of plan as to when, where, and what she can and wants to eat, as well as places that can accommodate her, especially if she's still suffering from any morning sickness. In addition to avoiding exotic foods she can't eat, you should probably avoid excessive walking, bungee jumping, helicopter rides (BMP will be shaken, not stirred), and deep-sea fishing (motion sickness plus diesel fumes equals . . .).

Exploring Paternity Leave

Unlike most civilized nations and third-world countries, Americans have no paid leave policy when it comes to having a baby. While some companies have policies in place to allow mothers a civilized period of time to welcome their child into the world, dads have no such luck. So save your vacation days, and check with your employer's human resources department to see whether you have any chance to take an extended unpaid leave (if you can afford to take it).

Paternity leave is quite a nice little thing. You're indirectly asking your employer to give you paid time off to be with your new baby. In the executive office, knowing they have to pay you for some period of time, even though you're not ill and can still perform your duties, is probably as popular as poop sandwiches, underwater stock options, and male secretaries.

Needless to say, most companies don't have overly extravagant policies. They may run from eight to twelve weeks on average, and often you'll receive some portion of your compensation, but give up any bonuses or special pay you may have received. Do your homework and see what you should expect.

If your boss is reasonable, it may be a good idea to sit down with her and see what her general attitude is about the situation. This is important; in some cases you may discover how sympathetic an ear your boss has when it comes to matters of the family. There are bound to be a couple of occasions where you'll need a little extra time to help with Junior, and it's good to gauge just how that will be received. As with anything, the more planning the better. If you have extra vacation time available, you may want to bolt that onto your leave. If grandparents are interested in coming to lend a hand, plan around that as well. There's no sense in having triple coverage when double coverage will do. Extend for as long as possible the time someone will be at home with the new mom— she'll need all the help she can get. She isn't going to be feeling 100 percent, and caring for and adjusting to this new child will prove to be slightly overwhelming for her and for you. The longer someone is there to help, the greater chance for all involved to maintain their sanity for a longer period of time (but not forever). So plan your time away from work in conjunction with any and all of the trustworthy help you can get.

One father is more than a hundred schoolmasters.

—George Herbert

Making Sense out of Every Dollar

Man, these babies can be expensive! But this is not the time to feed your inner CEO and look at your child-to-be with an eye on its ROI. Even so, you do have to plan for the baby's expenses, just like you've planned everything else. Disposable diapers alone cost about $100 a month. Now, you need to feed and clothe this baby, because child-labor laws prevent you from sending babies out into the workforce for another few years. So there are a couple more things you'll need to budget for:

- **Special furniture, appliances, and transportation needs.** Car seats, high chair, changing table, and stroller. Don't forget to throw in a bouncy seat and toys. Oh, and the high-definition baby video monitor, complete with night vision! Try getting some of these items second-hand, as hand-me-downs from friends and family, from garage and yard sales, from Craigslist, or at consignment shops. Check the Consumer Product Safety Commission's and manufacturers' websites to make sure anything you've purchased used hasn't been recalled for containing lead paint or deadly metal spikes. Maybe you can space out your purchases and purchase items you won't need right away further down the line.

- **Baby clothes.** Didn't we just splurge on maternity clothes? Crap. Still, with all the stores out there, the law of averages means some baby clothes will be good enough for your baby. Another option is to find less expensive, "gently worn" clothes. This is code for used. Consignment stores can help clothe your newborn on the cheap. Unfortunately, working against you is the fact that these kids tend to grow. So as their size changes, you'll need to buy new items. Depending on where you live, you may also need to buy seasonal items. Don't forget, you'll be in a perpetual cycle in which Baby outgrows his clothes and needs new ones. If you're considering having more kids, box this stuff up.

- **Education.** Feeling like a go-getter? It's never too early to put aside education funds. More parents are sending their kids to private schools across the United States. Oh, and don't forget college. The cost of college tuition is rising faster and faster. The home-schooling trend seems to have some momentum these days, as parents save money. If private school is too expensive and the public school is unacceptable, this may be your only choice. (Just make sure your child is exposed to other children more frequently than once a month, or your son will end up being that guy in the office who doesn't respect personal space and whose breathing is actually audible during meetings.)

- **Life insurance.** Do you have life insurance? If something happens to you, do you want your BMP to face a difficult choice such as going back to work, taking on a second job, or finding another breadwinner? At least discuss this one with your BMP. There is no magic formula. Simply figure out what exactly you would want the life insurance proceeds to cover, and calculate how much that would cost. If you want your BMP to have a paid-off house, some spending money, no debt, and Junior's college all taken care of, I hope you're a skinny nonsmoker. Oh, and God forbid something happens to Mom, but you'll want to have insurance on her. You would be overwhelmed enough without having to take a second job at Red Lobster.

- **Activities.** Assuming you care about your creation and want her to actually have some sort of balance in life, you'll want to find some activities your child can

take part in. Gymnastics, tennis, karate, music les-
sons: your child is a blank slate. It's okay, however, to
allow for some unstructured play time (wait, can you
plan unplanned play time?).

- **Vacations.** If you want to test your gag reflex, price
out an elaborate family vacation. There's a reason
Disney allows you to book far in advance and make
payments. As you add kids, you end up with bigger
rooms and more mouths to feed.

It seems like you may have to hock your jewelry as well
as one of your kidneys to be able to afford Junior and everything that comes with having a baby. You just might have
to. The latest numbers compiled by the Families and Work
Institute show that more than 75 percent of married couples
have both parents in the workforce. Fortunately, parents
have an uncanny way of making it all come together. Most
of this magic comes from parents giving up stuff for themselves. It's *okay*. What did your BMP need with that new
Coach purse, anyway? It doesn't hold things any better than
her old one.

Budgeting for Single-Income Families

If you want to make a go as a single-income family, here
are a few tips:

1. **Don't give up retirement savings to make it happen.** Although those 401(k) dollars haven't been
growing lately, don't think about discontinuing
retirement-savings contributions as part of your plan
to become a single-income family. You don't want to
count on social security alone, do you?

2. **Make a strict budget.** It's pretty pedestrian advice, but let's face it: most people don't have a written budget. Know what your fixed costs are every month (car, mortgage, cell phone) and whether there are any places where you can cut back.

3. **Practice.** Before one of you boldly marches into your boss's office and declares yourself free of his shackles of slavery, make sure this new financial picture is sustainable. Have the paycheck of the spouse who is going to quit working put into savings for a few months, and try to make it happen on a single income. Then you'll know whether this is a realistic option for you.

Finding a Pediatrician

You'll want to choose your pediatrician before you bring your child home. You'll find out that babies need to go to the doctor often—even more so if they're going to be in group child care. Their immune systems are limited, and they can catch just about any germ that's out there. Before this happens, take the time to select a doctor for your new baby. (Guess what? We get another fun list!) Here are a few of the criteria you can consider:

1. **Does the doctor take your insurance?** Or, if you have an HMO or PPO, is the doctor in your network? Incompatible insurance is obviously a deal-breaker in my mind. Bringing a baby to the doctor every couple of weeks is very expensive, and that's what insurance

is for. This is almost like when you were looking for a college; you started with, "Can I get in?"

2. **Meet the pediatrician ahead of time.** Good pediatricians set aside time to meet with parents-to-be. Many times the personality of the caregiver is the deal-maker or deal-breaker—how she acts, the way she handles your toughest questions—these are all intangibles that you have to sit through an appointment to really evaluate.

3. **Hours of operation and answering service.** Babies often wait until the middle of the night to have problems. They're just testing your love. You'll want to know whether your doctor's office has an answering service that will call you back, no matter the hour. This can be pretty handy: the doctor on the other end of the line can guide you through that all-important decision, from "This is no big deal" to the other extreme, "Get to the nearest emergency room right away."

4. **Check out the office.** Make sure it's somewhere you can see yourself bringing your child. Not every hotel has a five-star rating, after all.

5. **How difficult is it to get an appointment?** This is a simple exercise. Call in the morning, ask for an appointment, and see what they say. If the answer is "A week from Wednesday," maybe this office has taken on too many patients. You can also ask how many patients the practice serves. More than thirty patients per doctor in a day gets into puppy-mill territory. Sometimes these busy offices will give you a recommendation. If you go to your first and second appointments and have to wait an hour past the

scheduled time, that's another sign that the practice is overstuffed with patients. Some offices have nurse practitioners, who are often easier to schedule with but lack the MD after their names. They can usually get the job done on day-to-day sniffles and fevers.

6. **Check out the doctors in the practice.** How long have they been in business? Did they get their medical degrees online or at a school you've actually heard of? You want a doctor who knows the most recent research and keeps up to date. As with your BMP's obstetrician, most pediatricians practice in groups, and you won't always be able to get in to see your primary caregiver. You'll want to make sure the reserve players are as good as the all-star you picked out.

Just as there are some signs that you might have found a good pediatrician, there are several signs you may be on the wrong track. Just a few of the more obvious ones:

7. **As the doctor leans over to pick up some trash,** his white coat slides open, revealing a T-shirt that states: "My PhD stands for Party Hard, Dude!"
8. **The fine print on his diploma reveals that he graduated from Doctorsrus.com.** His minor area of study is listed as kegology.
9. **While being escorted back to the examination room, you overhear the doctor telling someone how he applied to the FBI to be the dedicated physician for all female agents.** "Then," he continues, "I could tell everyone that I was always right, FBI really does stand for Female Body Inspector!"

10. She enters the first appointment smoking a cigarette, and then offers you a glass of wine while you wait.

Finding a Day Care

It's common for both parents to work. So unless one of you is able to perform masterfully at your job while caring for a child at the same time, you'll need to make arrangements for your baby's care while you two parents earn a few dollars.

Many dads are not quite in touch with the reality that you need to do this well ahead of time. All of the quality day-care providers—and even some of the average day-care providers—in your area may have waiting lists. So you need to get out there and scout these places out. If you find one that meets or exceeds all of your requirements, you'll find yourself doing everything within reason to secure your child's spot at that location. You may even find yourself slipping the director of the facility a C-note to help things along. Oh, come on, just kidding (as far as you know).

As you and your BMP talk to enough parents about their day-care providers, you may begin to sense that most of them are making the best they can of this situation, and you'll usually be correct. Any decent day care is very expensive, but when you go for an on-site visit, it may leave you underwhelmed, or simply whelmed. Many of the "teachers" may have trouble with grammar, selecting a flattering hairstyle, and remembering to brush their teeth on a regular basis. This is not the house of dreams you envisioned leaving your little angel at for long periods of time. So right off the bat, you're attempting to reconcile the cost with the quality of the personnel.

It's time for another one of my lists! I know you're excited:

1. **Quality of care.** This is the most important piece, and I talked about it above.
2. **Location.** Location is extremely important; hence its place near the top of the list. If one of you travels for work, pick a location near the parent who doesn't. If a situation arises, such as when your child gets sick, you can be there at a moment's notice.
3. **Certification.** We all know that government-run programs are about as effective as having Charlie Sheen as your AA sponsor. But certification is a must-have on your list. You've got to think to yourself, "If they're not smart enough to get government certification, do I really want them in charge of my child?" Most of the facilities you're likely to consider will have this, and should.
4. **Caregiver-child ratios.** The ratio is important. If you have any imagination, you can see how taking care of one single infant will be a challenge. Now multiply the required amount of love and attention by ten, or more realistically, multiply it by fifteen. So if they have fifteen infants to every caregiver, you can imagine how well that may work. A good ratio in the infants' room is three or four babies to each adult.
5. **Open-door policy.** Can you stop in anytime you want to see your child? If you stop by unexpectedly, you can learn a lot by seeing the teachers when they

don't know you're going to be there. Many parents will only use facilities that have webcams installed in the rooms so you can view your child whenever your heart desires. If for some reason the facility doesn't allow parents to pop in, this would have to be taken as a red flag.

6. **Cleanliness.** This seems obvious, but check anyway. With all of those little people running around eating, drooling, and pooping, the place can get dirty and germ-ridden fast. Good caregivers stay on top of things. It's a bad sign if they don't. I'm not suggesting you secretly use a swab on the welcome tour and get it sent to a lab for analysis. Just use your eyes. And nose.

7. **References.** Ask the day care to provide some names of customers who use their services. If you want to be tough on them, ask for a few names of people who no longer use their services and interview them.

So once you do all your homework, how do you decide? There is no foolproof methodology. Some simply look at what they can afford. Others look at the various costs versus the benefits. If you can, stay around the facility for a few hours, and you'll get a feel for whether the staff really cares for the children. That plus the location and price should be the ultimate criteria. A quick tip: many employers offer an account that allows you to pay for dependent care with pre-tax dollars. Every little bit counts!

Birth Announcements

Unfortunately you can't just post the following announcement on your fantasy football message board: She did it! The
baby popped out. It's a boy, and he's hung like his father.
Everybody's fine!

To most guys, this probably covers all the needed information, but it's not going to make the grade. You're going
to drop more cash than you feel is reasonable to announce
your offspring's arrival into the world. Unfortunately, this
requires trips to some sort of store created out of most men's
nightmares, as well as lengthy discussions about paper thick-
ness and quality, in-depth analysis of font type and size, and
the difference between Cotton Candy and Cherry Blossom
paper samples. As your frustration builds, refrain from these
common responses:

- I don't care.
- Just pick one.
- I'm leaving.
- Where's the nearest bar?

Like many things in life, sharing these feelings will feel
good in the moment, but there will be payback later. Just
strap yourself in for several hours spent dedicating yourself
to differentiating between shades of light pink or blue. As
the price per announcement climbs, you'll want to fight
back and cross those third cousins off the recipient list.
Don't sweat it. Maybe the force will be with you and those
long-lost relatives will give you some of the best gifts.

One night a father overheard his son pray: "Dear God, Make me the kind of man my Daddy is." Later that night, the father prayed, "Dear God, Make me the kind of man my son wants me to be."

—Anonymous

Do I Really Need to Buy Her a "Push" Gift?

First and foremost, let's define exactly what a push gift is:

Push gift (n). A ridiculous concept created by women to begin a trend in which they receive a gift in exchange for carrying a baby to full gestation. Their hope is for this to become a common practice the whole world over.

Okay, so this definition is sarcastic, inflammatory, and for the most part, meant to be in jest. Looked at one way, a push gift lets men acknowledge the pain and sacrifice women go through to carry and birth a child into the world. But on the other hand, there is no "emotionally scarred for life" gift for men or a "you've been wrong for nine straight months" gift to reward us for making it through pregnancy. If you and your BMP decided to procreate, it really wasn't a question of "Okay, who is going to carry this thing? Honey, are you sure? Thanks for stepping up to the plate."

So my advice is this: if the gift comes from a good place in you, then go for it. But if you happen to pick up a vibe about how the cost of the gift will be evaluated as a measure of your love, or if your offering will be compared to what So-and-So got from her husband, then at least try to get store credit when you return the gift.

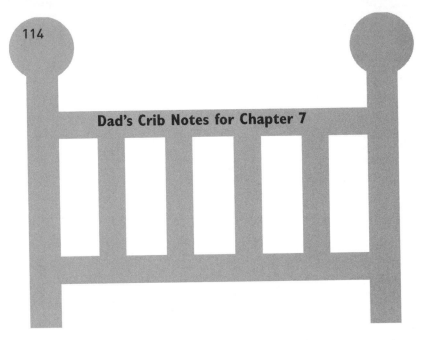

Dad's Crib Notes for Chapter 7

- There may be some fun things the two of you want to do as a couple before the baby comes.
- Always get the doctor's permission, but consider a nice vacation.
- Make sure to check with your employer's human resources department concerning paternity leave. You may need to plan your vacation accordingly to maximize the time you can stay home after your baby is born.
- It will be important to plan out a new monthly budget for the family. Make sure to include any new expenses such as day care.
- Family vacation destinations will most likely change, as will the cost!
- Take this time to research and select a pediatrician for your child. Start with a list of providers covered that are by your insurance and are located near home, and then go from there.
- If both parents will be returning to work, it will also be important to find a day-care provider.

- Birth announcements are an important way to formally notify important people in your life about your new addition—just don't break the bank!
- It's up to you whether you want to follow the recent trend of getting your BMP a push gift.

CHAPTER 8

Babywatch

As you near weeks 38 and on, you'll be a vigilant member of what the media would name Babywatch. While it's not as stimulating as *Baywatch*, which exists so viewers can ogle beautiful lifeguards as they run down the beach on TV, Babywatch consists of staying in constant contact with your BMP, texting her to see if she "feels" anything happening in there while the two of you are apart, and generally being a pest. But your efforts are not mistimed: Although only about 4 percent of moms give birth on their due date, about 98 percent give birth during weeks 38 through 42.

Although only about 4 percent
of moms give birth on their due date,
about 98 percent give birth
during weeks 38 through 42.

For your BMP, the rest of the way home is going to get pretty uncomfortable. It's guesstimated that she'll gain about a pound a week for the rest of the pregnancy, and because she's roughly the size of a barn, she'll have a harder time moving around and will suffer more aches and pains.

What's Junior up to? Your new baby's all-over fur is falling off, and regular hair is beginning to really grow, including eyelashes. The natural coloring is beginning to fill in. Your baby's lungs are starting to become all grown up, and although I do not recommend trying it out for fun, he can breathe air if necessary. Your baby is able to open and close his eyes. Regardless of race, creed, color, or religion, his eyes tend to be dark gray. The real eye color doesn't fully show until after the birth.

Some babies begin to suck their thumb at this point and can cry in the womb, which is amazing, as it seems akin to crying underwater. Junior can even be scared by a loud noise, which is also pretty amazing.

Also, the little person drinks amniotic fluid and pees in the womb. While slightly weird, it's totally natural—and it may even help prepare your child for swimming in public pools when they get a little older than, well, zero. It's no coincidence that your child is developing immunities to mild infection through Mommy's antibodies, which cross the placenta.

Because your child is growing so rapidly, the womb is beginning to feel like a studio apartment in Manhattan. The baby's movements may press against your BMP's internal organs, causing many bathroom trips if it's the bladder the baby is pressing against, and pain if it's a rib.

As your baby's knees get tucked up close, you can probably figure out where the term "fetal position" originated. But of course, as all children of the 1980s and fans of classic Patrick Swayze movies can attest to, nobody puts Baby in the corner. At least not for long. Your baby is getting ready for delivery and may "drop"—that is, sink down into your BMP's pelvis to get into launch position. Some doctors will start giving weekly exams at this point, checking to see whether the cervix is moving forward, whether it has begun to efface (stretch out), and whether it's starting to dilate. If in addition to this, he asks your BMP if she's happy with her relationship with you, well, that's a different story entirely.

The Freak-Out

Somewhere around this time, the phenomenon known as the "parental freak-out" occurs. Sometimes this "what the hell were we thinking?" moment is brought on by the more visible signs of pregnancy, such as the growing belly of your BMP. It can be stressful for everyone. It's a feeling so strong, you'll want to press the Panic button on your car key to see if someone will come to help you. That loud sound that won't go away is you panicking about becoming a parent. Common thoughts include:

- "How will we pay for her education?"
- "I'm not ready for this!"
- "All of my cash is going to be spent on diapers and baby chew toys."

What you're really asking yourself is, "Will I be a good parent?" and also, "Will I lose my sanity?"

Unfortunately, the magic formula for parenting was lost long ago. Little known to you, your BMP will probably be having these thoughts as well; she's just handling it better. Exhaustive study of stories told by fathers around poker tables, bar rooms, big-screen TVs, and outdoor grills has shown that women seem to be naturally programmed to handle this whole thing with a little more grace and confidence than you.

Sherman made the terrible discovery that men make about their fathers sooner or later . . . that the man before him was not an aging father but a boy, a boy much like himself, a boy who grew up and had a child of his own and, as best he could, out of a sense of duty and, perhaps love, adopted a role called Being a Father so that his child would have something mythical and infinitely important: a Protector, who would keep a lid on all the chaotic and catastrophic possibilities of life.

—Tom Wolfe, The Bonfire of the Vanities

The best thing to do is talk to your BMP about the game plan. You may have different ideas on what's important, and it's best to figure these things out ahead of time. Even if you lose every coin flip on issues you disagree about, at least you'll know what's headed your way. So take a deep breath, relax, and go watch an episode of *Cops*. It will make you feel better about yourself and your prospects as a parent.

Packing a Bag

Before there's any chance of delivery, it's important for you and your BMP to pack a bag to take with you to the hospital. You will need a few items besides a change of clothes and a toothbrush. Let's get some insight into what a well-prepared hospital bag might be holding:

1. **The birthing plan.** This document contains all the decisions you made back when you were calm, cool, and collected. You gathered all of the information, considered the options, and decided what you want. So when all hell breaks loose, you'll be ready for anything.

2. **Let me entertain you.** You need to bring stuff to do. If the hospital room doesn't have a CD player and a DVD player, make sure your iPod makes the trip, and consider bringing along a portable DVD player. Books and magazines can keep you occupied. Photo albums may be a nice way to reminisce. A laptop is a must in today's world, and don't forget your Blackberry if you're a workaholic. Just don't get caught Tweeting during the birth. I can see it now: "@johnpfeiffer—Dude! Just cut the cord!!!"

3. **You're getting sleepy.** Dads usually get sleeping accommodations roughly equivalent to a sleeping bag shoved into a corner of the tent, so prepare accordingly. If there's anything you can bring to help

yourself sleep comfortably, make sure it's in the car. Some dads I know have gotten away with only sleeping at the hospital for one night, but 75 percent of those men are now single.

4. **Hi Gene!** Toothbrush, toothpaste, deodorant. Also, don't forget your common over-the-counter ibuprofen and other common medications. These items don't come with your deluxe accommodations, and like any good hotel, they charge triple in the gift shop.

5. **Femme fatale.** Remind your BMP to pack any items that you're embarrassed to buy at the local grocery store. She'll know what she needs.

6. **Baby items.** Important! Pack the car seat and a new outfit for Junior. Ah, and your first pack of diapers.

7. **Don't forget camera and camcorder.** You and your BMP may want to record portions of the big event. Other portions had best remain private.

8. **Contact information for relatives, parents, and in-laws.** You want some of these people at the hospital. You really don't want them in the room during the action, because let's face it, you don't invite them into every aspect of your personal life. You can have them in early, when nothing is really happening, and make it clear that when you give the signal, they're expected to clear out. Then when everyone has their act together, you can bring them back in, and as a special privilege, one of your lucky family members can be sent out to get you and BMP a decent meal. Who says in-laws are useless?

Dissecting Advice for New Dads

During this exploration of pregnancy from the male perspective, I've often mentioned the advice that's out there.

Plenty of websites for pregnant women give advice to dads. Why are these lists always written by women for men? We don't attempt to write "Dealing with Women's Issues" articles. This is probably because we couldn't handle it. So here are some common tips, and my reaction to them:

Tip 1:

Babies aren't that fragile, so don't be afraid of yours. Ask your partner, a nurse, or your own mom how to hold the baby if you're concerned.

My take:

This one is on target. We're not really known for our gentle holding of anything, except, possibly, for breasts. Plus, as single men, we've always left the room in any situation where it appeared we might be required to hold an infant and symbolically ran away from settling down. We have no experience.

Tip 2:

If your BMP and the new baby are bonding like crazy, and you're wondering, "What am I, chopped liver?" talk about it.

My take:

This is one where the Men's Union just needs to get the word out to women. During pregnancy, we often feel left out. But I don't really see a sweeping challenge to the male ego if we approach our partners and say, "Gee, honey, I'm feeling a little left out." So this tip is on target.

Tip 3:
Those hormones don't stop after birth, so your partner will have ups and downs after the baby is born. Be supportive and listen to her concerns. Educate yourself about postpartum depression and seek help if needed.

My take:
I agree. I'd add another point: these things may also happen to Dad, but it's not always as visible because our bodies don't change during the pregnancy. We can get postpartum depression, too, but it may be harder to see. The assumption is that if men don't discuss their feelings, everything must be fine. That's not always true. So keep a close eye on yourself, and on your BMP, and if you notice emotional changes, speak up, or get yourself some help.

Tip 4:
Express your pride in her breastfeeding efforts, and help her deflect negative comments about it. Take a breastfeeding class with her.

My take:
Who are these people giving negative commentary about breastfeeding? We know it's healthier for the child. As for the breastfeeding class, if the video is anything like birthing class, there is no way. It seems like a slight stretch to ask a guy to say, "I am so proud of you, honey!" when he sees his BMP breastfeeding the newborn. I just don't think

many men are going there. I'm also not sure what we're being proud of. Maybe wait until she's putting on a dazzling parenting display that you could never pull off. This will happen. Then let her know she's a good mother. This just seems more genuine than complimenting her lactation technique.

Tip 5:

You can do everything but breastfeed. Remember to help around the house. Don't let your partner worry about the housekeeping. Take on more chores so she can get extra sleep and recover.

My take:

This one gets tricky. Everyone is taking on a lot of extra responsibility. My best advice is to prepare yourself emotionally, as if the pilot had just announced, "We're headed for some turbulence." This is a tough time for everyone, and both parents need to pitch in and give it their best. A friend of mine makes sure to tell new dads: "Hey, the big secret is the first year sucks." It's not true for everyone, but it happens. Also, these articles are often written by women for men. Something smells fishy here. It seems like there may be a conflict of interest. It's a little bit like me starting a lingerie advocacy group. A sure recipe for disaster is for either parent to feel like they're getting the short end of the stick. Discuss your feelings and expectations, and get to know hers.

Tip 6:

Ask for help. Know who can give it.

My take:

Definitely. Having the phone numbers of doctor and babysitter in a predetermined place is a must. I'm not sure lactation consultants are as critical.

Pick and choose. Much of the advice is very sound and should be followed. On the battlefield of information, you need all that you can get. But despite all of this, make sure you get a few tips from a father you know who will shoot you straight. Getting all of your relationship advice from women feels a little like getting your wife a male doula. He might have all the proper information, but how could he really know what it's like? You could do it, but you probably wouldn't.

Preterm Labor

This is a buzz kill. It can happen any time from week 20 on. Any labor before a woman completes 37 weeks of pregnancy is still considered preterm. If your BMP actually gives birth prematurely, the seriousness of any complications is correlated with how early the baby arrives. The earlier it is, the more serious. Symptoms of preterm labor include:

- More than five cramps or contractions in an hour
- Pain during urination
- Backaches
- Bright red blood from the vagina
- A clear watery gush from the baby house

These are the most common, although there are others. Always know whom to call in these situations, and have your physician's contact numbers programmed into cell phones, posted on the fridge, or tattooed on your shoulder.

Your doctor may prescribe certain medications if preterm labor is a possibility for the mother-to-be. Outside of medication, staying hydrated is one of the better methods to prevent preterm labor. Dehydration can cause lower blood volume, which in turn increases the oxytocin levels in the blood. Oxytocin is the hormone that causes contractions, which can cause preterm labor.

Bed Rest

About one in five pregnant women get put on bed rest as a preventive measure. Basically, bed rest means spending pretty much every day in bed, all day. This may be for the last week or so of pregnancy, or it may be for a month or more. Generally it's prescribed for child-and-BMP teams who are at risk for preterm labor, when the child is not yet fully developed. It's also commonly prescribed for those who are carrying twins.

Just know that there are different flavors of bed rest. Sometimes doctors will instruct their patient to only observe partial bed rest, while other times it's so strict that a bed pan becomes necessary. The surprising twist here is that although it's still commonly used, bed rest may not help women who are prescribed it, according to some studies. So this is really going to be a doctor-by-doctor decision. Read up on the subject, always discuss with your BMP, and see what your doctor has to say.

The surprising twist here is that although it's still commonly used, bed rest may not help women who are prescribed it, according to some studies. So this is really going to be a doctor-by-doctor decision. Read up on the subject, always discuss with your BMP, and see what your doctor has to say.

Although it sounds like a vacation and an opportunity to create a "Top 100 Movies of All Time" list, some women think of bed rest as bed *arrest*. To most of us working stiffs, what we hear through our burnt-out ears is that the doctor is giving your woman an excuse to live out your dream. She has been *ordered* by the doctor to lie back, relax, and catch up on that *Mad Men* marathon you've both been meaning to tackle. It would not only be irresponsible for you to ignore the doctor's advice, it would be downright *unsafe*.

But what seems to happen is that after a couple of days of being restricted to bed, these women start to go insane. They feel isolated from the real world and from people in general. They don't talk about how great bed rest was for them, or how they felt recharged and ready to re-enter their lives. No, on the contrary, they tend to talk to each other about how they can *survive* bed rest. Men everywhere are still waiting to give this a try.

Let's look at what her situation is, and how you can help your beloved if she happens to be put on bed rest:

- **Line up her day.** If you're going to work, think about what she'll need while you're gone. Can you give her breakfast before you go to work? Make her a little lunch and put it in a cooler beside the bed, and make sure water is readily available. Make sure she has a cell phone within reach. If caring for her will make you late at the office, plan for that as well, or have a friend you can call who can cover for you.
- **Make sure she's busy.** While she can't begin the marathon training she had hoped to start, she can still do a lot of things while on bed rest, such as online baby-gear shopping and research, with a laptop. The worst part of bed rest seems to be the monotony and feelings of isolation. If your woman has some goals to work for and achieve, it can make her feel more engaged with the world.
- **Keep her entertained.** Supply her with books and magazines. Suggest little projects she can do, such as keeping a pregnancy scrapbook or just about anything positive to break up the monotony of lying in bed and waiting.
- **Misery loves company.** A perusal of the web will show that there are now online communities for women on bed rest. It's a good idea to encourage her to communicate and commiserate with those who are really feeling her pain in a way you can't.

Fetal Distress

This is pretty much exactly what it sounds like. Something is causing a problem with the baby. Likely causes can be medication, infection, or, if it happens during labor, the

induction process. An irregular reading of the baby's heartbeat will be the best indication of fetal distress.

Meconium

What is meconium? It's baby's first poop, a thick, green,
tarlike substance. Please note that despite the description, it
cannot be smoked, even in California. Usually this crap stays
in your baby until after the birth, but about 30 percent of
babies have a moment on their amniotic throne before birth,
and that can cause problems. The meconium gets into the
amniotic fluid and is in turn ingested by the baby. In extreme
cases of high meconium concentration in the amniotic fluid,
your caregiver may even inject sterile fluid to help dilute it.
As your BMP passes her due date without giving labor, the
chance of some meconium getting into the amniotic fluid
rises. Another problem is that your baby may inhale it, and
that can cause serious problems after delivery. If this happens,
the doctors will suction out Baby's lungs and throat (to ensure
that your baby isn't full of crap, like his dad).

Umbilical cord around the baby's neck

Do we really need to discuss this? Just the visual image
alone is enough to depress me. The fact is, as the baby moves
around in the uterus, the cord can wrap around the baby's
neck. About one-third of children are born like this. So it's
not as rare a situation as we first thought.

The best thing to do is to first find the doctor you want
to work with and to discuss the risks of the above situations.
These are big scary problems, and you need a doctor's perspective to understand your risks.

Okay, let's all shake it off. I thought it was important that you got that information. So far the pregnancy has been a snuggly love-fest, and you've taken to calling each other nicknames such as Pookie, Snook-ums, and Honeybunch. The weird thing is, you find yourself into it. You even heard yourself call her Angel Cups, and you meant it! What the hell is going on? Don't worry, the pregnancy process is about to take it up a notch. Let's get to where the action is: her cervix.

I Saw the Sign, and It Opened Up Her Cervix

If your BMP begins to feel any or all of these symptoms, it may be time to grab the hospital gear, review your birth plan using those cramming skills you learned in school, put on your nurse's outfit, and head for the door:

- Regular contractions that get closer together, while lasting longer and becoming more intense
- A trickle or gush of fluid from her vagina
- A backache that keeps better rhythm than you do on the dance floor

Things are getting very real now as the projected due date creeps closer on the calendar. You should check with your doctor before taking any long trips by land, sea, or air. Doctors, who are like regular humans except that their brains are larger, have different opinions on the subject. If you and your BMP have been experiencing problems during the pregnancy, the doctor is more likely to withhold the hall pass, especially if the trip is noncritical.

It's not only trips by land, sea, and air that you need permission for. Yes, even the most personal of areas, your love life, has been changed by the baby. At this point in the pregnancy, if you plan to take a trip to the bedroom, you must in effect check with your doctor first. You may not have ever thought you would utter the words, "Is it okay for me to make love to my wife?" to another person, but it's the safest course of action. Your doctor may blurt out, "Oh, and it's okay for the two of you to go at it like rabbits." Then you're saved from asking.

Encouraging the Baby to Come

When a pregnant women gets to a certain point in the pregnancy, say, somewhere around 38 weeks, if the baby is healthy and ready, her attitude becomes one of, "Let's get this thing out of me!" It's understandable, as she has lost her figure, her ability to eat normally, and of course, her mind.

Let's take a look at some old wives' tales about how to cause that baby to evacuate. While some of these may help, I don't recommend trying them without talking to your doctor first.

1. **Taking castor oil.** This remedy has been around forever. The theory goes that if you drink castor oil, it will cause the muscles in your body to contract and get the ball rolling. There are many, many, instances when this has worked for women, and it seems to be effective mostly for those in early labor. But there are also many reports of women throwing up and get-

ting diarrhea but no labor. The verdict is that this is unpredictable at best.

2. **Eating spicy food.** No concrete evidence exists that eating spicy foods will work as a way to induce labor (this also applies to eggplant Parmesan; I hear this one often as well). There's a chance that spicy foods help produce contractions by irritating the bowels and dehydrating the body. Spicy foods also increase production of a hormone that can begin the labor process. More importantly, there is not really any downside to trying this option. Well, she might get an upset stomach, but nothing too drastic.

3. **Massaging pressure points.** This is one method that has pretty much been proven to work. The only problem is that if the person who applies the acupressure doesn't know what they're doing, they can do some real damage. Don't even fool around with this one. Let this method remain an "ancient Chinese secret."

4. **Walking.** Here's another natural method that works for many, but not for everyone. If you see a very pregnant woman determinedly walking the mall or hiking up and down steps, you'll know what she's up to. This method also has a side benefit: even if it doesn't induce labor, it will often help the baby drop, or move into labor position.

5. **Having sex.** This might be as old as being pregnant. Sex causes the body to produce oxytocin, which causes the uterus to contract. Nipple stimulation can also produce oxytocin, but to a somewhat lesser degree.

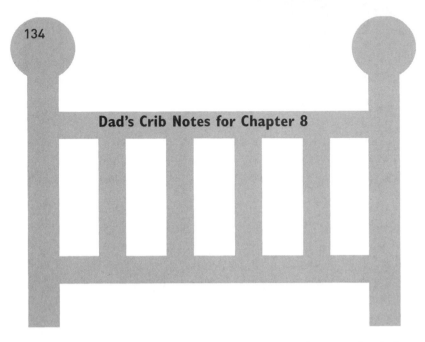

Dad's Crib Notes for Chapter 8

- It's almost time. Are there any preparations you've left to the last second? Because we are there already.
- If you haven't felt totally overwhelmed yet, it may happen around this time, when you're so near the actual birth. Don't worry, though; parents always seem to find a way to make things work.
- Pack a bag with everything you will want and need for your hospital stay. Put some thought into it now, while there's still time.
- Not all advice for new dads is created equal. Seek out a dad you trust and respect, and talk to him about the fatherhood experience.
- If your BMP is placed on bed rest, it will be up to you to take extra good care of her. Although bed rest seems like a relaxing prescription, it drives many pregnant women crazy.
- Be familiar with the most common difficulties that can arise during pregnancy and labor. Make sure to discuss them with your BMP and health-care provider. Know

what your plan will be if these unfortunate circumstances arise.

- Make sure to know the signs of labor, although your
  BMP will probably know right away.
- There are some common old wives' tales concerning
  kick-starting the labor process. Make sure your health-
  care provider knows what you're up to before you take
  matters into your own hands.

CHAPTER 9

The Birth:
Special Delivery

Birth: the event of being born. I especially like this definition because childbirth is an event. Friends and relatives may travel from miles around to see the beginning of a new life. It is an event because it is something special, something we have only partially been able to figure out. It is an event because there is an element of the unknown, and all hell might break loose. Finally, it is an event that will be happening soon to you and your woman!

Methods for the Madness

By now, you may have the birth plan finalized, in ink, and even laminated, with copies for all of the doctors and nurses. But even so, let's examine different methods of the event of childbirth.

Mother Nature

Occurring less frequently these days is the old-fashioned way of giving birth. Nature does its thing, and when the baby is ready, it comes out. You know that your BMP's water may break in an unexpected place, and as you near the due date, maintaining a constant state of readiness becomes a pain in the ass. But when it happens, the adrenaline rushes and out the door you go!

To Drug or Not to Drug

One of the major decisions you and your BMP face is whether she'll take pain-killing medicine during labor. Actually, it's her decision, because unless she punches your face during labor to help you share the pain, there's really only one person who is feeling pain, and it's not you. An epidural is the most common form of medication. The actual drugs involved are usually a local anesthetic coupled with a narcotic. This will relieve the pain while allowing her to remain totally conscious during labor. The main advantage to doing this—besides getting a narcotic—is, well, lack of pain. The dose can also be instantly modified if the location or severity of the pain changes. This method keeps the amount of drugs that reach the baby to a minimum. Lastly, if she needs to have an immediate C-section or other surprise surgical procedure, the anesthesia can be adjusted accordingly.

As always, there are some downsides to the whole drug situation. You may feel like it's not a natural way to deliver. That's up to the two of you. Also, after painkillers are administered, many hospitals will require women to remain lying down. Epidurals also have a habit of slowing down labor and can reduce feeling during the pushing stages. In some cases, the dosage may not be correct, resulting in less than full pain relief. Side effects from the epidural can include itchiness and nausea. So, including the reduced feeling from the waist down, she may have an unexpected potty break. Men aren't allowed to say this out loud, but let's face it: we're lucky we don't have to go through this.

Induction

Induction is the process by which your medical-care professional attempts to jump-start the childbirth process. This is most often attempted by introducing medications: a drug such as Pitocin that helps labor start will enter your BMP's body through an IV, and drugs such as Cervidil, which ripen the cervix, are introduced vaginally. These medications should cause the labor process to begin.

Make sure the two of you have had a conversation about induction and whether you're for it or against it. As the days go forward and still no baby, your doctor may suggest inducing labor. The risks include the possibility of stronger contractions. This can increase discomfort (an understatement) for your BMP and elevate health risks for the baby. Increased risks include:

- More intense pain for your BMP during labor
- Baby ending up in the NICU (neonatal intensive care unit)
- Need for a C-section
- Various degrees of complications associated with preterm labor. You are, after all, evicting Junior before Mother Nature has given your baby his get-out-of-the-womb-free card.

When it comes to birth by induction, it won't be quite as action packed as the deliveries you see in the movies. Actually, it can be a little anticlimactic. Your doctor says the bun has been in the oven long enough and it's time to take that thing out. Much like your local handyman, she'll give you a date and time range such as, "We will complete the miracle of life on Friday, October 18, from 6 to 9 P.M., and then fine-tune your HD." As long there aren't any emergencies, the doc will give you the call from the bullpen to come to the hospital. You slowly and patiently bring your travel bags and arrive in no particular hurry. The medical team puts your partner—and unfortunately, not you—on drugs to get the ball rolling.

Tweeting Dos and Don'ts

Don't forget the fun possibility of Tweeting the experience for your Babywatch followers. Because you will be delirious, sleep deprived, and generally not thinking clearly, here's some advice. Please **do not** Tweet any of the following:

- "She's either pregnant or she ate a baby."
- "They just paged my wife's ankles to the delivery room because we couldn't find them."
- "She's currently attacking her food with the intensity of a wild boar."
- "Just judging by belly size, I'll make this call: Surprise triplets!"
- "The doctor told her to push, but she's not really trying."
- "I think we can answer the question right now: We got milk."
- "When I find out who the father is, I'll kill him."
- "I feel like I'm at a private screening of Big Mama 2."

- "I going to go rub the Buddha for good luck."
- "I cannot believe she wimped out and got the epidural!"

C-Section

Certain circumstances call for the doctor to go ahead and, for lack of better verbiage, bring the baby into the world by cutting open your BMP's abdomen and lifting the baby out. Slightly gross. Some women prefer to do this to help maintain their appearance. They're either planning on leaving you very soon or they're extremely vain.

Most frequently this procedure is performed because of pregnancy complications, and if your BMP has a C-section, it's likely that subsequent deliveries will be performed that way as well.

Here are some common reasons why a C-section is performed:

- **The labor process gets stuck in neutral. This is called "failure to progress."** The baby seems ready, Mom and Dad are ready, but nothing is happening. Up to this point, the labor has been all anticipation and no follow-through, like Clay Aiken's singing career or an Adam Sandler movie. Perhaps the baby's head is too large to pass through the birth canal. Anyway, this is the most frequent and least problematic of the C-section situations.
- **A more problematic situation is one I alluded to before: your baby's oxygen supply has been reduced.** Either this or a dramatic change in the baby's heartbeat can cause your doctor to recommend

a quick surgery to get the baby out of there. Nothing like a little excitement to spice up the delivery.

- **Location, location, location.** It's possible your child has entered the birth canal in a less-than-ideal position. You simply cannot leave some things in the hands of a baby. The baby might be breech, or entering the birth canal feet first. This often happens with multiples. Babies can also get comfortable in the horizontal position and cannot be moved into the correct launch position. A C-section procedure can fix these thorny problems.
- **Placental abruption can occur, when the placenta detaches from the uterus (not yours, Daddy) before labor gets underway.** Placentia previa can also occur—that's when the placenta covers the opening of the cervix. If either of these situations occur, it will be safer for the baby if a C-section is performed.
- **Also, your baby may have health problems that make this type of delivery safer.** If your baby has or may have conditions such as spina bifida or extra fluid on the brain, your doctor may make this recommendation.

So if C-sections are so handy, why don't we deliver all babies this way? The main reason is that, like all surgeries, there are risks involved. Of course, surgery involves general cutting and so forth, and either your BMP or the baby can get accidentally injured. C-section babies have an increased risk of having breathing complications. Mom also faces a number of risks, including endometriosis, or an inflammation of the uterine lining; additional bleeding compared to traditional birth; urinary tract infection; and a three to four times greater chance of blood clots. In emergencies, it helps to have knowledge of the procedure up front. Being informed will reduce stress and fear of a C-section delivery if there's a complication with the delivery and the decision must be made immediately.

Besides being informed, you can take a few additional steps to get ready if you're so inclined or think this may be a real possibility for you. This may include—you guessed it—another blood test so the doctor has all the blood-matching information available in the unlikely event that your BMP would need a blood transfusion caused by blood loss during the C-section procedure.

Assuming everything goes well with the C-section, there are still some post-surgical considerations. Mom may not be allowed to lift anything heavier than a baby, and will need lots of help. Coughing, sneezing, or laughing at your wonderful jokes can cause mild pain or possible bleeding. Just so you know, most C-section patients will not be able to have doctor-sanctioned intercourse for at least six weeks. It's way down on the list in importance, but I thought I should break it to you now.

After the delivery, by whatever method, the health-care staff will examine the child and make sure everything is functioning correctly. And unless you're living in a country with a heavy government where they're already determining whether your child will become an Olympic hero or an assembly-line worker, you should receive your child back shortly, even if she's genetically destined to become a gold-medal winner on the vault.

Bad Things, Man, Bad Things

So there are a couple of things that happen during birth that you are most likely not prepared for. There isn't sufficient warning, either, because they're just too utterly indescribable, or perhaps people—and men in particular—are too embarrassed to discuss them, or, most likely, it's a diabolical plot that gives those who have already been through the experiences described here something to laugh about. So, for the first time in print, we'll detail these mysterious events:

- **Color and odor of the water breaking.** When the baby is ready to show up for the party, the amniotic sac ruptures, and the amniotic fluid—aka "water"— sometimes gushes everywhere. If your BMP's water decides to break, with any luck at a dinner party at the home of a friend you secretly dislike, the doc or midwife is going to ask you about the color and odor of said water. Because your natural reaction would be to rush over, stick your whiffer right up close, and breathe deeply, right? Of course your next reaction would be to take note of the color. "What do you think, hon? Kind of a translucent cadet gray? Or closer to oyster?" Needless to say, the description in question is not solely for the doctor's amusement. Based on your detailed description, the doctor can hope to discern whether there are any potential problems going on.
- **Somebody is going to poop in her pants.** Isn't this just what you wanted to see? There is a strong possibility that you, your BMP, or little Junior will

make the delivery room a makeshift throne. You, because you're scared as hell; your woman, because of the extreme amount of time and effort spent pushing. Make sure you're comfortable with the people in attendance. Tell your sister not to bring her fiancé; he might never recover. Between the many reports of record-setting gas with a chance of poopiness, you're in for a memorable experience. In the event that you escape the scenarios listed above, the baby will be the culprit. Your baby has been taking in nutrients, and to celebrate their arrival, some babies like to get that meconium out of their system.

- **Cutting the cord.** We've all heard about the figurative cutting of the cord. When a friendship doesn't work out, or a boyfriend or girlfriend needs to go, we've all bitten the bullet and ended the relationship. But this cutting of the cord is literal. You're in the delivery room, having made it through the obstacle course of delivering a child, feeling happy and relieved in the seconds immediately after you've first seen your new child, and you're hoping you're in the clear and everyone is happy and healthy.

The doctor turns to you and offers you a medical device that's the equivalent of scissors. It's as if you're being tested. Are you man enough? Can you overcome your natural programming, which tells you to recoil, feeling you may cause harm to Mommy or your new child? From someone who has been there, I cut it, but I do not judge. Mostly because I am squeamish and feel ill at the first sign of blood.

Fetal Monitoring

Whew. Fun stuff. Labor and delivery can be like making sausage or seeing Kirstie Alley in a bikini: not all that pretty. Still, we're not through yet, so let's keep going.

During labor, you might see a beltlike contraption looped around your BMP's belly. This is for fetal monitoring, which allows your doctor (or, more likely, the nurses) to keep vigilant watch on your child, his heart rate, and how he's handling the contractions. Some hospitals do not use the belt and do a manual check at regular intervals, say every fifteen minutes. If they use continuous monitoring with the belt, and if things are really slow, don't be afraid to encourage your BMP to remove it to, say, go to the restroom. This will be a good dry run to see if anyone is paying attention up at the front desk. (Disclaimer: They may get mad at you, so I'm joking here. I think.)

One other method may be used, and in the interest of full disclosure, I'll tell you about it. If your BMP is—how do I say this—full figured, it may make it hard to get an accurate reading. In these cases, the doctor may use internal fetal heart-rate monitoring. Here they actually attach a monitor to the baby while Junior is still in utero.

If the fetal heartbeat shows a rhythm or pattern that causes the health-care staff concern, they may instruct your BMP to change positions, or they may give her more fluids. A more serious pattern could cause the doctor to consider other delivery methods; the most common would be an immediate C-section.

Once you arrive at the hospital, you get settled in and go through the process. It's a little maddening because the hospital staff generally acts like they're delivering a pizza, but it's okay for you to get excited.

Role-Playing During Labor

If you've taken on the mantle of "labor partner" for the delivery of your child, then all of us other guys are really proud of you. This title implies more than just telling onlookers when they may enter and when they need to ske-daddle. If you're considering a home birth, this role is even more involved.

So what *is* your role during labor? Why do I always pic-ture a guy doing these weird Lamaze breathing exercises? Well, if you've been involved in the process from the begin-ning, going to all the classes and appointments, then you're right on track. If you're reading and trying to stay informed about pregnancy and delivery, kudos—you're doing a great job. You most likely picked up a lot of what you need if you've been doing all of the above.

A quick Internet search will show articles with advanced labor-coaching techniques such as, "Don't answer your cell phone or text" during delivery. Hmmmm. Methinks some-one had a bad experience with men. Also out there is advice like, "Refrain from needless chit-chat that can annoy her" during this magical moment. How about some tips that are actually helpful for men and not tinged with poisoned estrogen?

1. Guys, remember, you may not feel like you're doing a whole lot. But by being there you're supporting your partner and showing solidarity with her.

2. It's okay to be nervous. She's nervous. Encouraging her during the contractions and delivery is one of the most important things you can do.
3. Pray together if you are so inclined. (Screaming about blessed feces does not count.)

In the days immediately following the birth, it will be important for her to know how much you love and care for her, and that she is still beautiful. I encourage you to give her a map with Tennessee cut out, and tell her, "You're the only 10 I see."

I guess it's time to discuss with reverence the miracle that is childbirth. When you stop to consider how smart and efficient nature is, it really is amazing. A single, determined, sperm dodged all of the various dangers as if it were in a microscopic game of Frogger, and made a final triumphant leap to its destination. This small, fertilized egg finds its own way to be implanted in a uterus. In this tiniest of blueprints is carried the information to grow everything from ten fingers and toes to the complex human brain. Eventually this growth takes the aforementioned single cell all the way to a fully formed baby.

So as you stand there in shock as you watch your child enter the world, take a quick second to realize how amazing this whole thing is. Unfortunately, these minutes of rapture and amazement must end. But before you know it, you and your BMP will be alone in a recovery room at the hospital with huge smiles on your faces that won't go away easily.

Post-Birth Hospital Dos and Don'ts

Okay. I lied to you. I told you I was going to abandon you after the birth. But I've grown fond of you as the pages have turned, and it just wouldn't be fair to leave you now. I have a soft spot for new fathers because I just think they are so wide-eyed and on edge, like newborn puppies. I can at least stay with you until you get the baby home.

Let's take a look at your best strategy for navigating the post-birth part of this journey. As I mentioned earlier, they're going to do some funky things with Junior. It's okay. As long as you're not giving birth in a third-world country where they're estimating your baby's worth on the black market based on your and the mother's appearance, the doctors are generally just checking everything to ensure that Junior is in good health and checking whether there are any superfluous tests they can justify to soak the insurance company out of a few thousand more dollars. Some of these tests include a hearing test, Apgar test (which judges the baby's overall appearance and breathing), PKU test (which detects an important enzyme or its absence), a blood test to determine the baby's blood type, and, depending on where you live, perhaps a few more. Your baby will also howl in indignation as the shots are administered: a Hepatitis B shot and Vitamin K. Someone will also measure your baby's weight and length.

After the medical staff gives you the thumbs-up, they generally flop the baby onto Mommy and clear out. If the grandparents are present, sober, and not ex-cons, let them hold the baby. You most likely will need their free caregiving services in the future. Often all the attention goes to Baby, while Mom, who just went through the equivalent of passing an eight-pound watermelon, sits all alone. If you plan on sticking with her, or if you just want to keep the child-support payments slightly lower after your divorce, hold her hand and give her some love. Your child doesn't even know who you are right now, so she won't hold it against you.

As for the kind of love you haven't had for a few weeks and yearn to give your BMP, sorry, Charlie, it's not going to happen for a while yet. Unless you're strictly a north-side daddy, you just witnessed another human emerge from the same zip code you used to use for your sexual pleasure. Not to kill your dream, but things on that side of town are going to need a few weeks to get back to normal after your love child passed through. Your gratification is once more on hold and is quite possibly, um, in your own hands.

You've made it through the birth, God willing, with a healthy baby who will be happy until you ruin his life. We can worry about that last part later. Now that the main event is over, it's time to navigate the all-important post-birthing process. Please listen carefully. First and foremost, let the baby go to the nursery as much as possible. Erase the guilt by reminding yourself that you will need every second of sleep you can muster to be at the highest alertness level in the care of your bundle of joy. The hospital staff is professional and equipped to handle anything that comes up, and you probably are not. So let Junior hang out with you and your BMP for a few hours at a time, but then send Junior to the nursery. This may be your last chance to sleep for more than four continuous hours for the next few years, so enjoy it.

Next, you'll be receiving a visit from La Leche League. Be afraid. Be very afraid. It's unconfirmed that these people are the modern offshoot of the Nazi party. *Do not* by any means leave your partner alone for this experience. These people are only slightly less dedicated to breastfeeding than suicide bombers are to their cause. They will use *any* means necessary to achieve their goal, which is to get the mother of your child to breastfeed. They will use guilt as their primary weapon. As their fanatical website is happy to inform you, breastfeeding leaves no carbon footprint. Take their information for what it's worth, and if they get too aggressive, leave a carbon footprint on their ass as you kick them out of your room. You and your child's mother, but mostly your child's mother, will make a decision in the breast-versus-bottle controversy.

Start Spreading the News

In a post-delivery world, you'll want to get the wonderful news out. All of those donors—otherwise known as friends and relatives—who contributed by purchasing carefully selected gifts will want to be in the know as soon as possible. News spreading will usually come in two separate waves.

The first wave is close friends and family, who will want to be informed of the miraculous miracle of life as soon as you know about it. If you want to spare yourself many finger-numbing dials, and further spare yourself the repetitive Q&A, I strongly recommend you hire a service to leave a message in an impersonal, robotic voice: "(BEEP). This is not a telemarketing call, an unwanted solicitation, or a collection agency. James Earl Pfeiffer was born October 18 at

7:43 A.M. and weighed in at . . . ." If, for some odd reason, you find this approach too impersonal, I guess you could do what everyone else is doing and start a Facebook page for everything birth related. Although it's not as bizarre as the telemarketing-like recording (although still fun), you do get to play God by carefully considering whether you want to accept Aunt Judy's "friend request" because, frankly, her gift sucked. Plus, you get to post information and pictures without really having to speak or interact with anyone. Who doesn't love the digital age?

The second wave comes when you inform people outside your close friends and family. This includes third cousins and Uncle Bernard. Of course, you will also need to notify your bosses and coworkers. Someone such as your boss's assistant can handle the internal dissemination of the news of a successful birth. One simple call or e-mail, and everyone gets the word. This is good because it proves to your boss once and for all that you weren't faking this pregnancy thing for a little extra vacation time, and everyone from the lowly interns to upper management will know about the new addition to your family.

Back to those pesky friends and family. They just won't give up, will they? You will be required by social contract to create a birth announcement, created from an unflattering picture of your recently arrived child, whose face bears a bewildered look after being ripped from his or her home.

Papa's Got a Brand-New Life

Stick with me here: this is for your own good. Fatherhood is a huge change for men. After losing our virginity and winning our first legal wager for more than $5, it's probably the most transformational moment for us. Most guys never know what hit them. There they are, going along with their life, and then bam. The Fatherhood Smack-Down. Well, if you've made it this far, you deserve full disclosure.

There are three stages of a man's life: he believes in Santa Claus, he doesn't believe in Santa Claus, he is Santa Claus.

—Author Unknown

Becoming a father is both the most rewarding and the most challenging job you could ever sign up for. The pay is lousy, and the hours are roughly equivalent to all day, every day, for the foreseeable future. Fatherhood is one of the experiences in life that you cannot possibly prepare for. It's also one of those unique life experiences where there is no one right answer. There's no manual to outline what to do in certain situations. You have to make it up as you go along.

Are you ready for all of this? I know I had no idea what I was getting into. Maybe that was a good thing. During the pregnancy is a good time to start getting involved in your unborn child's life. A new member of your family is coming soon. Parenting is no simple matter. Whether you notice that the third-most-popular article on a pregnancy and parenting website is "Drinking Alcohol While Nursing" or you missed Tyra's special on "Soccer Moms Who Smoke Pot," you'll quickly get the idea that you're not the only one who feels overwhelmed.

Preparing to Play Dad

What have you done in preparation for this? Done any reading? Taken any classes? Do you have a plan? If you don't stick your nose in there and get involved, it will be easy for your BMP to run the show as you fade into the background. So take a few minutes to think about it. How are you going to make sure you and Junior bond? Planning to take your child on a special one-on-one scheduled activity is a great start. Mom gets a break and you stay involved. Seek out another father, or even *your* father, and see if you can learn anything.

What you're really getting to work on is worrying less about yourself and more about what your family needs. These needs may be somewhat mutually exclusive. You need to get that fancy sports car you've dreamed about. The family needs to get a larger car to transport everyone. You and your BMP need some alone time to rekindle the bow-chica-wow-wow. The baby needs to be fed every couple of hours, and rocked and held in the middle of the night. It's an extremely tough row to hoe, but it needs to be done.

Take Care of Yourself

The books she's reading are about her, the baby, and then her again. Who's thinking about you? I hope it's your BMP, although she has a lot of changes going on as well. One simple recommendation is to make sure you're taking care of yourself. Know what you need to take care of yourself, to keep yourself engaged in your life as a father and husband, and to have balance with your work and social life (just kidding—your social life is over). Having a child can be very stressful to your relationship. The child-centric families of today have helped develop the dissatisfied spouses of tomorrow.

As your beloved surfs the web, she'll come across many women who've written advice articles for their sisters. It's a mixed bag of advice at best. But there's a definite subsection of these articles, blogs, and opinions that are about as unbiased as Fox News. They often promote women for women, with a not-so-subtle undercurrent of men being the lesser of the two parents. Some go as far as to characterize men as clueless in general. (So I guess I should cancel "Stogies and Poker" as the baby-shower theme?) You're often placed at the lowest spot in the pecking order by the "experts" and "advice givers" out there. Does a man put his family first? He must. But one of the best ways to be a strong father and partner is to make sure you're taking care of yourself as well as your family. It's walking a tightrope and requires some retraining (6 A.M. run, anyone?), but it *can* be done if you put in the effort.

You and Your BMP

Having children seems to have a way of shining a harsh light on any problems you and your BMP might be having. If you argue about money, things will only get tighter. If you argue about frequency of sexual interest, the two of you are only going to be more exhausted and less interested. And if you can never seem to have enough time in a day to get everything done, the time will only get more precious. This stress can lead to problems if it's not managed correctly. And there's a uniquely male problem: we need to find out exactly who this new person, "Dad," is—this person we've become.

For new dads, the hardest part is finding the correct role to play. Breadwinner? Mr. Mom? Clueless father? It won't be easy, but you have to find your role and define for yourself how you're going to take part in your child's life. You're

going from being defined as someone's son to being someone's father. Don't think it's as easy as pouring your coffee
into a World's Greatest Dad cup and you're ready to go.

Fatherhood is losing half of your vocabulary because

you cannot swear in front of your kids.

—Doug McDougall, parent and nerdy engineer

Let's face the facts, men. We find ourselves in difficult
times. Men are torn between worlds. Our traditional role
has been pretty solidified for many years. The majority of
the time we're still expected to earn an equal or greater share
of the money to support our growing family. That's how
men take care of their family. But at the same time, our
involvement in parenting has grown. This is a good thing.
We have greater enjoyment of our families as well as deeper
relationships with our children. But there are very few men
for whom the lesser financial role is an option. In many people's minds, stay-at-home dad translates to unemployed dad.
A father with a lower-earning job can be seen as a lesser
man in some way. Not only does society at large promote
this viewpoint, but we ourselves place this stigma on each
other. So let's take a minute to redefine what it means to be
Dad. Next time you meet a man whose primary role may
be caregiver, remember that it's okay. Because if we're to be
judged, as a father and a man, by the number of zeros on our
paycheck, I have demands. I want immediate reinstatement
of fedoras, the Rat Pack, lunch martinis, and weekly poker
night, complete with cigars and gin and tonics. I personally
prefer Thursdays.

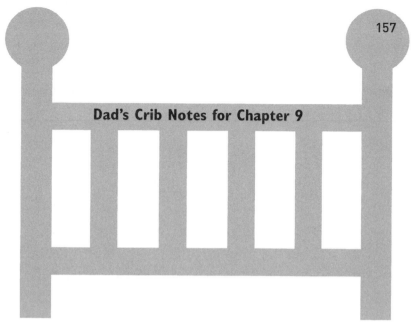

Dad's Crib Notes for Chapter 9

- Read up on all the birth options. Learn about all the different delivery methods there are.
- Daddy, you have a big decision to make: are you going to cut the cord?
- After the birth, there are a few things you can do to make everything a little easier. First and foremost, let the trained professionals care for your child in the nursery so you and Mom can get some well-deserved sleep.
- Once you return home, you will want to get right on those birth announcements.
- As we have discussed, your life is about to undergo many changes. Coming home with a new baby is the sure sign those changes are starting.
- To be an effective parent, sometimes you have to make sure you're taking care of yourself.
- Just as you need to take care of yourself, you should strive to keep a strong relationship with your BMP. It's your love that brought this child into the world, and it's your love that will make sure the child is raised correctly.

PART 4

The Fourth Trimester

Whew! You made it. You made it through all the trials and tribu-
lations of pregnancy. Now what? Well, first, go get your car out
of the parking garage. It's time to go home. Make sure for the
103rd time that the car seat is installed properly, and head out.

Your time to stay with your BMP and Baby will, with luck,
last for a few weeks, allowing you to bond with your child and
have a transition period before returning to work. This will give
you some experience in the life of your child. You can learn
how to change diapers, maybe give the baby a bottle, and
most importantly, rock her back to sleep in the middle of the
night while you're only half awake yourself. Your skill set will
definitely be expanding, although these skills will not show up
on your resume.

That nursery you worked so hard on together will finally
have a resident. All the purchases and gifts you had momentarily
forgotten about will be put to the test. Soon you'll learn how
to perform many tasks one-handed, as there is usually a baby in
the other hand. You will also reconsider the importance of sleep
in your life, as the baby will need to adjust to a set schedule. All
of the changes we've helped prepare you for are now very real.

CHAPTER 10

Taking Junior Home

You made it! You're now the proud owner of a brand-new baby. And it's a trying time, to be sure. After you've stayed at the hospital for your insurance company vultures' approved two or three nights, it's time to go home. The postpartum area of the hospital is a halfway house for the mentally insane. You get a few days in an artificially controlled environment to ease into your new life. For new parents, these artificial controls include the ability to send the baby to the nursery while you grab some much-needed sleep; trained personnel available around the clock at the push of a button; and cable TV. For new parents, coming home is the next step into the madness that is society at large, where you lose the doctors and nursery, but possibly have family and doctor-prescribed Percocet to keep you relaxed.

As the daddy, you witnessed with squinched-tight eyes as your baby came into the world. Even if you closed your eyes all the way, simply hearing the screams and imagining passing a human out of your body will lead you to logically conclude that the new mother might not be feeling too well.

With that in mind, it's your job to screen the visitation privileges of both friends and family, based on your BMP's tolerance for them. You may secretly relish the opportunity to tell her disapproving parents that, sorry, they just can't come over today. The newest mom on the block will have some residual pain, and the house might not be presentable, and the two of you might not be presentable, but nobody cares, they just want to see the baby. Don't be afraid to screen your phone calls or turn off the ringer. A sleeping baby will become a very valuable thing in your life. We'll get to this more in the "Visitation Policy" section below.

Your other job during this time is to try to introduce your child to some kind of reasonable schedule. Babies tend to be happier and easier to wrestle when they maintain a regular eating and sleeping schedule. But brand-new babies may not care what your schedule is, so you have to train them. The sooner they adapt the better.

You may be introducing the family pet to your new child. This can be easy or quite tricky. Some pets may consider themselves the family baby and become jealous. Others may see themselves as protectors of the baby. And most cats could simply not care less. Consult your vet for the best methods to use when you're integrating your new family member.

Real-World Bonding

Your new family member is going to do his best to test the limits of your sleep deprivation, as well as your tolerance limits for certain scents. Because you'll be pouring your heart and soul into your efforts, you might as well love the person you're doing it all for. For some, it can seem as if there's no bond at first. Don't panic: it will come with time. Others hit it from the jump and are head over heels from the minute they see their baby. Here are a few tips on bonding with your new child:

- **For boys:** This one is easy. What says "bonding" like beers and wings at the local Hooters? Unfortunately, you are about twenty-one years too early with this plan.
- **For girls:** This one is a no-brainer as well. Just give them your credit card and point them to the nearest mall. Just as unfortunate: they will probably chew on it, and you'll get in trouble for giving the baby a dangerous toy.

So what do you do? The answer is different for everyone. Letting the little one lie on you and nap is always a crowd-pleaser. Playing and feeding (often intersecting with one another) can be fun—if messy—activities. Take her for stroller walks and to movies. Simply incorporating her into your lives a little at a time is all it usually takes—that and the guilt and fear of knowing that you can screw up this kid all by yourself. Parenting is such a difficult job that it's best tackled by two people, or at least one extraordinary individual. If you stay at it, you'll feel connected soon enough. But, until then, go ahead and take at least one activity and make it your time with Junior. Maybe you're the almighty bath giver. Perhaps you make watching football on Sundays your time with your child (but be prepared to miss a good bit of the game). The old-school "let Mom do everything" is all but gone, and you need to get some baby skills. Even if you start small, you and your child can start bonding, and you can progress from "the guy who gives me baths" to "Daddy."

After the initial rush is over, your life begins to change rapidly. Most studies focus on Mom's postpartum depression, but remember, guys, we can fall prey as well. Just remember the signs for you and your BMP, and seek help accordingly. Some of the most common ones include feeling overly sad, having no energy, overeating or undereating, feeling no connection to your child, and, the most serious sign of all, telling your friends that you've lost your mojo. Make no mistake: this is a life event that will change you. You may have had certain hobbies or activities that were once tolerated by your BMP, but once a baby is on the scene, they'll be discarded faster than a girlfriend who brought an extra 100 pounds back with her from her summer vacation in Europe.

Where Do I Fit In?

This is a tough question. Let's review the situation:

You're at a point at which you're expanding your family from two people who care for and love one another to three people. This third person, whether because he's a helpless infant or he's just extremely lazy, cannot care for himself in any way, shape, or form. So that takes time and effort away from you and your woman. You and your partner can't pour as much energy and effort into loving one another as you used to. In addition to time and effort, resources are expended to make sure that Junior has every advantage possible. With this reallocation of effort and resources, certain things become unrealistic for the two of you as a couple.

Maybe your thing was to plan last-second getaways. Maybe you visited your university annually to catch up with old friends. Many of these activities become problematic. The logistics grow more difficult: you'll suddenly need a grandparent or two to agree to come watch your child.

The place of the father in the modern suburban family is a very small one, particularly if he plays golf.

—Bertrand Russell

So the situation is that you have diminishing time, effort, and resources. Kids become the priority. What's that old saying? "You think you know, but you have no idea." This is one of those situations. Everything from meals to bedtimes to the type of car you drive will be affected. Your new boss wears a diaper and doesn't have much in the way of hair, or fine motor skills, for that matter.

Do you know what's the strangest thing about all of this? You're going to love it. When I say you'll love it, I don't mean it's a cut-to-the-front-of-the-line ride to eternal bliss. But I guarantee that unless you're a distant relative of Burgermeister Meisterburger (this will make more sense when your child is around age two and it nears Christmas . . . thanks), you won't be able to help but feel a swell of love and joy when you look at your child. It's so unique, it doesn't even fade over time. So while there can be an adjustment period that lasts for different people from between one minute to one lifetime, you can have a special relationship with your child that stays strong and vibrant.

Now we've all looked up and realized that we're holding hands and singing. Boy, this is awkward. While we recover, let's get back to your pole position. By "pole position," I'm speaking of the family totem pole. You know what I'm going to say, don't you? No, you really don't. You thought I was going to say everything you want, all of your interests, are going to come in dead last. But this is a common misconception. To quote Vince Vaughn in *Swingers*, you are all "growns up."

You (should) have a job, and at any time, you can move your priorities to the front of the line. The twist here is that you and your BMP *volunteer* together to put the interests of your children before your own. That doesn't mean that the two of you can't arrange responsible supervision for the kids and sneak off to Pigeon Forge for some hanky-panky in a Champagne glass–shaped hot tub. It doesn't mean there won't be times when you'll want a two-seater convertible. Doesn't mean you won't struggle with it and mess up sometimes. But by doing this as a team, a unique team that likes to explore each other's bodies, you can make this work. *That's* where you fit in.

Visitation Policy

After giving birth, depending on what exactly happened in that delivery room (please don't make me remember), Mom is not going to be looking for every friend, family member, or nosy neighbor who has baby fever to come parading into your home and put their grubby hands on Junior. She may not be feeling like herself, and sleeping will be a priority for both of you. To further lower your tolerance for the parade of well-wishers stomping through your house, just imagine your reaction as your mother-in-law's friend proceeds to tell you how sick she's been feeling as she holds on to your little bundle of joy. Babies' immune systems are not fully developed, and they are apt to catch any illness they come into contact with. So between your woman's feeling not quite right and your child's being in a slightly fragile state, you feel a strong urge to disconnect your doorbell and post signs like "KEEP OUT" and "BEWARE OF DOG" and be done with the entire situation.

It's okay to make the people who want to come bearing gifts wait a few extra days. If there are persistent "helpers" whose mission in life seems to be to annoy you until they get to help and feel better about themselves as people, let them. In fact, if they fit this bill, size them up. Where do you think their strengths and talents lie? Asking the busybody neighbor to prepare a dinner is a common practice. Having any nonrelative get your oil changed or run errands for you is probably going to the extreme. However, going to this extreme and making it painful may mean that they never stop by again, so you may want to give it a try. This may take the form of telling them the coffee they picked up for you was prepared incorrectly, or asking them to go back to the restaurant because something wasn't cooked just right. This should hold them at bay for a while, even if your reputation suffers in the 'hood.

But there might be a select few whom you *do* want to come for a visit, assuming they're in good health and didn't forget to wash their hands after their Swingers Club road cleanup that was held this morning. This is where you come in. Now it's your turn to act like one of those bouncers at the swanky clubs. Put a velvet rope across the front door.

Hit the gym seven days a week, shave your head, and forget how to smile. Heck, wear a fake CIA earpiece if you really want to get into your role. Now you're ready to effectively monitor the riff-raff who are hoping to gain access to your exclusive club.

You can pick up some points with the new mom for handling the traffic flow and looking out for her and the baby.

Consult with your BMP to establish the hours of operation, and how many guests are allowed through the rope at any given time. This strategy will help you accomplish a couple of goals while keeping you in observance of the fire code. It will keep your child from being overexposed to anyone who may be sick, and will also allow you to keep control of your schedule. You'll learn that being on a consistent schedule is one thing that keeps a baby happy and healthy. Also, you can pick up some points with the new mom for handling the traffic flow and looking out for her and the baby. One caveat though: not everyone will be thrilled or even respectful of you for turning them away from Club Baby. Just be prepared for an aunt or neighbor to be offended when you tell them the baby is sleeping and no, you will not awaken her just for their viewing pleasure.

Bottle Versus Breast

We're going to kill a little of the drama here: experts agree that breastmilk wins, hands down. Breastmilk contains living white blood cells, as well as digestive enzymes. Your baby can get an immune-system boost from breastmilk too. Formulas simply cannot match this unique natural blend, no matter what the commercials say.

But here's where a couple of real-world issues come into play. If your situation makes it impossible for your child to be on breastmilk, then formula it is. Also, let's face it: Mom has an awful lot of say in this decision. If she doesn't want to breastfeed, for whatever reason, you're going to have a tough time making her do differently. So unlike those at La Leche League or some extreme mothers who shoot disapproving looks as you make formula for your child at the mall, you won't be judged on these pages. I can't find any study that links all high achievers in their respective fields to having been raised on breastmilk. Another potential plus is that with formula feeding, Dad can be more involved so it's not all on Mom. Here are some quick feeding tips:

- Newborns can only take maybe one or two ounces in a sitting. Their stomachs just aren't that big.
- Baby can actually be overfed. The doctor may advise you that Junior has a "formula belly." The signs are usually large amount of spit-up after feedings, and very frequent bowel movements.
- If your baby isn't gaining enough weight or seems to cry frequently, you may want to try feeding smaller amounts more often throughout the day.

That's really all you should need to know to get through this one. Oh, and if your BMP does decide to breastfeed, breast pumps cost about $200. Enjoy.

Daddy . . . Nooooooo!

Believe it or not, some new fathers actually make mistakes. The usual mistakes men make are not knowing their own strength, overdressing for the occasion, and being too good at listening. But once you become a father, you may make additional mistakes. Because we're not used to making these, I will cover some of them for you in hopes that I can help you avoid them:

- **Being a know-it-all parent.** Parenting styles are bound to be very different, and will in some bizarre way be based on the way you were raised and what you liked or hated about it. Because you and your BMP had different experiences, you're going to have different opinions on how to handle certain situations, and different priorities. Taking a my-way-or-the-highway approach isn't being a man, it's somewhere between being insensitive and being a jerk. Since this isn't something baby-less couples often discuss, you're liable to walk right into this one.
- **Going old-school.** You know who you are. You're this close to telling her to do chores and cook your dinner while wearing lingerie. You're the man, and dammit, you will do what you want. This act gets old three times as fast if she's working. And when I say

three times as fast, I mean she gets sick of it in four minutes instead of the usual twelve.

- **Ignoring Baby's crying.** Do you tell BMP to go make it stop, or let out a fake snoring sound? Always making her suffer through the middle-of-the-night baby duty, as Bryan Adams informs us, "cuts like a knife." But in this particular instance the only person it "feels so right" for is you and your selfish but well-rested soul. These really difficult parenting jobs need to be shared, and discussed. Parents can go from super teammates, where they are happily shouldering the load, to pissed and bitter, where they think they're being taken advantage of.

- **Hooked on a feeling.** How are you feeling, big fella? As I warned earlier, it's important for both of you to check in and make sure there's no depression creeping in. Men are especially guilty of not expressing themselves. If you have a bothersome thought roaming around that thick skull of yours, make sure you let it out. Don't wait for her to see smoke rising off your head to realize you might actually be thinking.

- **Master "listen versus fix."** Women are complex. Apparently they originally hailed from Venus. Sometimes they want you just to listen because they're frustrated about an issue. Other times, they're actually telling you to step in and fix their problem. Which is it? Just as women suffer from PMS, it says here we can begin to blame our confusion on our monthly bout with CMS, or Clueless Men's Syndrome. If I solve this puzzle, I will be more in demand as a speaker than Jack Canfield at the Campbell's soup corporate retreat. Until then, it's an art form, and talking about it together is the best advice I have.

Letting Grandparents Lend a Hand

Grandparents and in-laws can be either a helpful resource or a cause of stress when it comes to their grandchildren. Grandparents, and grandmothers in particular, cannot resist a newborn baby and will throw themselves at your mercy to get some special time with their grandchild. These attempts to monopolize Junior will be craftily disguised as attempts to help out the overwhelmed new parents, who are still adjusting to the exhausting demands of parenthood.

It *sounds* like a selfless act of goodwill, but, in reality, Grandmother (and possibly Grandfather) is watching you like a hawk and thinking about how you're doing it all wrong. If only she could get her hands on the little cherub . . . .

Never mind that you've attended parenting classes, read countless books on the subject, and have discussed all of the feeding, sleeping, and general safety concerns with your pediatrician.

Could these doctors and experts possibly know more than your mother? The answer is an emphatic *yes*, but you will never convince her of it.

I mean, your confidence in the grandparents was already shaken to the core on the multiple occasions when they offered your BMP a glass of wine during pregnancy. If this scenario sounds familiar to you, then all I can say is when you're asking the grandparents for help, *caveat emptor*. When it comes to helping out with their grandchild, your parents and in-laws can be very sneaky and conniving if they feel it's necessary.

For instance, you can tell the grandparents the correct position to lay down the baby to sleep . . . on its back, of course. Seriously, who hasn't heard of SIDS (Sudden Infant Death Syndrome) at this point? But it doesn't matter . . . there will always be that grandmother who, when you leave the room, will go in and turn that baby on its stomach because that's how you slept and you turned out just fine, thank you very much.

It may be necessary for you, as dad and Head of the Household, to intervene—not because you're worried about the crib death of your newborn, but because you're concerned about the safety of the grandmother who put the baby to sleep on its stomach.

Don't mess with a new mother—who's still raging with hormones—and her newborn baby. If the grandparents push too hard, they may get to meet Mama Grizzly Bear up close, and I am not talking about a Sarah Palin autograph session.

There are fathers who do not love their children, but there is no grandfather who does not adore his grandson.

—Victor Hugo

Still, grandparents *can* be a help. Grandmothers everywhere are begging for their chance to feed and rock the baby. Maybe it takes them back to a time when their breasts were able to defy gravity and turn heads. If you're functioning on two hours of interrupted sleep, their help gives you a nice opportunity to grab a much-needed nap.

This is what the chess match boils down to in its most basic form. The grandparents will wait you out until the baby pushes you to the point of exhaustion. That's when they strike, turning on their old-person charms and smiling kindly at you with their false teeth. You forget all of the things that bother you about them and give in to the siren call of your bed. But, no matter what feelings you harbor for the grandparents, just remember that their grandkids are one of the loves of grandparents' lives. It's that and Golden Corral.

Besides helping stave off the most severe effects of sleep deprivation, grandparents can help with the mundane household chores that are undoubtedly going to be neglected, since your main concerns will be caring for your baby, sleep (when you can get it), and an occasional shower. Unfortunately, someone still has to clean the house, cook the meals, and do the laundry. These are obviously the less glamorous tasks, so throw in some ample time with the grandchild as well, or their visit may not be as long as you anticipated. While the grandparents *say* they're there to help and will do whatever you need, what they really want to do is grab the baby when you aren't looking, jump in the car Pops kept running in the driveway, and take the baby home with them. And no, they probably don't think they need a car seat. (You didn't have one and you turned out fine.) Luckily, you can probably catch them on your bike, because they refuse to exceed their self-imposed 10-mph speed limit. Nobody knows why the bond between grandchildren and grandparents is so strong. Perhaps the grandparents just feel close to another human who has to wear a diaper.

Common Baby Myths

Grandparents love to give suggestions to their children about how to raise a child. The problem is, some of their advice is outdated. Here is a list of suggestions I have heard but wouldn't recommend:

Bad idea #1

If you want your baby to sleep through the night, put it to sleep on its tummy. At this point, I think we all know why this is a bad idea, but just in case you need a refresher, you should always put your baby to sleep on her back to reduce the risk of SIDS.

Bad idea #2

If you want your baby to sleep longer, or if Baby still seems hungry after he's has been fed, you should put some cereal in the formula or breastmilk. This is not recommended, because a newborn's digestive tract is not developed enough to handle solid food. Introducing solid food before four months may increase your baby's chances of developing food allergies.

Introducing solid food before four months may increase your baby's chances of developing food allergies.

Bad idea #3

You should give your newborn water in between feedings of formula or breastmilk. In reality, your baby is already getting all the water she needs from the formula and/or breastmilk. If a baby gets too much water, it can cause infant water intoxication, which can result in seizures. If your baby becomes dehydrated from vomiting or diarrhea, you should be giving her beverages especially made for rehydrating an infant, such as Pedialyte. Obviously, you'll be sure to ask your pediatrician about this first.

Bad idea #4

Don't let your baby "stand" or put pressure on his legs too soon or he'll be bow-legged. Okay, this is just a ridiculous old wives' tale that ranks up there with "don't allow a cat to be alone with a sleeping baby or it will smother it by sucking its breath." Most young infants will want to stand with support around two to four months of age. This is fun and exciting for them and is perfectly normal, and no, it will not cause them to be bow-legged. Unless their mom is Kirsten Dunst—but then it's just a case of genetics.

Your New Schedule

Perhaps I have mentioned that this child is going to change everything? Once the baby arrives at your residence, you'll have a new family member, a new schedule, and a new life. The fact that babies are not used to our world—or maybe the fact that they feel kidnapped from the home where they were perfectly happy—causes them to not really understand the difference between day and night. Add to the equation that babies are constantly peeing, pooping, or hungry, and you get the final result: babies cry a lot. Since they don't have any other means of communication, crying is their signal for just about everything. I'm sitting in my own poop?

Cry. I am hungry, and don't try to give me those infant sweet potatoes again? Cry. I'm bored? Cry. I think you understand. But if you tell me you don't, I might just . . . .

To be a successful father, there's one absolute rule: when you have a kid, don't look at it for the first two years.

—Ernest Hemingway

How exactly might this adorable but demanding baby affect your schedule? Let's do a quick comparison between a pre-baby and post-baby schedule:

Pre- and Post-Baby Schedule

Activity	PB (Pre-Baby)	PB (Post-Baby)
Saturday begins at	10 A.M.	6 A.M.
After a Friday night out, Saturday begins at	12 P.M.	6 A.M.
Average hours of sleep	8 hours	6 hours
Importance of naptime	It's on the list	#1 on the list
Nights out per week	1–2 on average	0–0.25 (1 per month)
Importance of your parents	Avoid them	Beg them to come over
Average bedtime	11:30 P.M.	10 P.M.

One of those infamous "studies" that was recently con-
ducted made the claim that on average during the first two
years of their child's life, parents miss an equivalent of 6
months of sleep. To be honest, I think they finally got one of
these things right. It's kind of like fraternity hell week for
two or three years. In my humble opinion, this is one of the
hardest things about having an infant.

Back on the Chain Gang

If you work in an office with enough people, you've
probably been around when someone else has had a
new child. You may have noticed that slightly rumpled
appearance and glassy look in their eye. It's probably
because they got their day started with a child who
decided to start their day at 4 A.M., and then this new
dad (or mom) spent a few hours of quality time getting their baby back to sleep, and rolled right into the
shower and then into work.

You may have also seen New Dad stupidly volunteering for assignments that required him to stay late or travel
overnight. This isn't due to his unwavering dedication and
passion for his job. The worst offender I had the pleasure
of working with was a recent father of twins. If there was a
legitimate reason to stay, he was there. This isn't to say he
was a bastard or that you should run for the hills, but more
to give you a feel for the degree of difficulty for what you are
about to attempt.

You might get a deluge of useless phrases like "work
smarter, not harder." But the reality of the situation is that
you'll be exhausted. Coffee and energy drinks will become

close friends of yours. The example given to me was that I would be constantly juggling, and from time to time I had to know which of the balls I could afford to drop without it breaking. Employment is most likely one of the last balls you want to drop.

Is It Sexy Time Yet?

Isn't it always? After the delivery, you'll feel euphoric. Like when your first issue of *Sports Illustrated* arrived with your free fleece jacket, but even better. If you followed the strategy discussed in the "Exploring Paternity Leave" section, you should be able to hang around the house for a few days with the family. You'll be caring for the baby, in awe of the baby, basically enjoying your new life as a dad. Eventually, you'll still be in awe and wonder, but you'll also be tending to other needs. You'll still need to sleep, eat, and exercise. As your new life takes shape, you may find yourself wondering, "When do we get to have sex again?"

Well, of course you're wondering this. You're still young, you're in love, and you're feeling happy about your life. The problem is that things may not be so cut and dried for your BMP. She went through a very physically demanding process, and, how do we put this, some of the hangover from delivery may delay her ability to express her love physically in the near future. The only way I know how to tackle this is to ask. But depending on the type of delivery performed, the time may vary. Were you paying attention? Did she have to suffer through an episiotomy? (If she did and you don't know what it is, dude. You need to pay more attention.) If she did, and you know what that means, you should also know this isn't something to mess with. Same with a C-section.

To give you some concrete idea of when your love may become real: most of the time it's not until the doctor gives the green light at the postnatal checkup, usually about six weeks after delivery. Again, if an episiotomy or a C-section was performed, all bets are off. Just assume it'll be more than the six weeks.

Getting a Babysitter

For the most part, grandparents make the best babysitters. For some parents, this just isn't an option. Moms and Pops may live too far away, or the two of you fight like cats and dogs every time their name is mentioned. Whatever the case, if you need a babysitter, here are some pointers to help you make a decision:

1. **Age.** Do you really want to hire a fourteen-year-old to be in charge of you baby? Most of them are still mastering the art of making their bed, and you're going to put a human life in their sparkly neon-painted-finger-nailed hand? Older babysitters have many advantages. They're more responsible in general. Plus, they sometimes have their own transportation.

2. **Experience.** This is strongly correlated to the age situation. Why would you want your child to be the one they make their rookie babysitter mistakes on? When you're talking about a sitter for babies, who can't exactly defend themselves or even tell on their

caregiver, it's best to get an experienced sitter with references.

3. **Certs.** I'm talking about certifications, even though it may make speaking to them more pleasant if they maintain fresh breath. Infant CPR is the most important, and basic first aid is a nice bonus.

4. **Pay the man.** What's the going rate for a babysitter these days? It's okay to ask them; they may recommend a pay rate. Although it's tempting to stick it to them if they leave it to your discretion, don't do it. Not everyone is as cheap as you are, and other parents aren't thinking, "If I give her $5 per hour, it's really like $7 pre-tax." The next time you and your BMP are headed out for the night, guess who's going to be without a babysitter?

Let's face it, good help is hard to find. Parents will not freely give up their number-one sitter just because you ask. Quality sitters get a lot of requests, so you'll need to ask early and often. You can explore the au pair/nanny situation, where you pay them a little extra to let you and your favorite girl go out on a Saturday night. Reserve them early, pay them well, and if you happen to get a college student who's home for the weekend to babysit for you, don't look at her that way, and everything will work out just fine.

Babyproofing

Have you babyproofed the house? If not, better late than never. Little kids will find ways to cause trouble in ways your adult brain could never imagine, and often times injuries ensue. Babies are curious little critters, and you'll need some new supplies to keep them from hurting themselves if you turn your head or fall asleep standing up. You need to go to the local baby mart and pick up some important items to take care of a few things:

- **Count all the outlets in your home.** You will need to purchase plastic outlet covers or sliding outlet plates. Most of the outlets are of the perfect height for a crawling baby to reach, and for some unknown reason, they're very inviting to babies.
- **Window blinds.** Take steps to secure the cord from window blinds out of Baby's reach. They're a choking hazard, even if you can't quite imagine it happening. Never place your child's bed near these cords.
- **Stairs.** Many families purchase baby gates. Different from the latest political scandal, baby gates are used to block both ends of the staircase to prevent a child from having a fall. They're especially good for when a ten-minute nap accidentally occurs.
- **Cabinets and medicine cabinets.** Once babies are mobile, it's game, set, match. They will open every cabinet they can, including ones that may hold cleaners, medicines, or other unsafe items. Make sure to purchase the babyproof clamps to keep all these areas secure.
- **Banister shields.** These are relatively new. They block the spindles of stair banisters or other areas. Babies can and will attempt to stick their head between the uprights, and shields will help prevent this from happening.

- **Kitchen.** Secure all silverware and other pointed objects, and make sure you check your cooking area. If you have accessible knobs on the range, there are, you guessed it, childproof covers for those as well.
- **Heavy furniture.** Any piece of heavy furniture, such as a dresser, that has a lower area where little hands can gain purchase needs to be secured with furniture straps. These secure furniture to the wall to prevent heavy furniture from being pulled over.
- **Garbage cans.** Besides the gross factor of going through the garbage, babies do not need to be able to get into any trash cans. Playing with trash is not pediatrician recommended, and if older babies pull on the top, they could get hurt. Many people put their trash can behind a babyproof door. There is also a trashcan that requires that you push a button on the back to open it.
- **Appliance cords.** Electrical cords or computer cords need to be secured or placed appropriately out of reach.
- **Fireplace.** Many babies have done some damage on these things. Buy some covers for all the sharp edges, and even consider blocking off the area if it can reasonably be done.
- **Carbon monoxide detectors and smoke alarms.** You need one carbon monoxide detector per floor, and smoke alarms in regular increments throughout the house, including one in each bedroom.
- **Breakables.** That ceramic clown Grandma gave you? If it sits on a lower shelf, then it's toast. Unless this is your goal (and it may be), move all these types of items up, up, and away from Junior. And if you want

to break something you hate and blame it on the baby, please do it safely.
- **Cage.** I highly recommend a baby cage. It's a small but growing trend. Seriously, sometimes it seems like this would be easier than all of the other steps. So even though baby cages aren't practical, taking baby-proofing steps is worth it. The guilt you would feel if something happened to your child would be horrible. You should at least know you made every reasonable effort to protect your child.

As a child of the 1970s, rereading this list makes me wonder how I survived past the age of three. We didn't even have car seats. It was very similar to the Wild West. On long trips, we folded down the two back seats in the station wagon and lay down. Somehow I lived to talk about it today. So, to answer your unspoken question: yes, some of it seems like overkill. And yes, the manufacturers are taking advantage of your parental guilt to turn a quick buck. But it just isn't worth it to save $50 on a baby gate, and while you're hatching a plan to escape to your weekly poker game with the extra fifty, your little one goes tumbling down, down, down. As in many scenarios in this book, grin and bear it.

It kills you to see them grow up.
But I guess it would kill you quicker if they didn't.
—Barbara Kingsolver

Now you're done. Junior is at home, on a regular schedule. You and your BMP have bonded with your child, and your life is nearing perfection. The hard work you've put in to transform your home into a baby-safe environment will finally start paying some dividends. Every stumble, bumble, and spit-up has been planned for, and you stand ready to drain your savings account to educate your child in today's questionable education environment, in which teachers make slightly more than janitors. Whatever your opinion on the topic turns out to be, just be ready to answer this question in the next six to twelve months: Should we have another one?

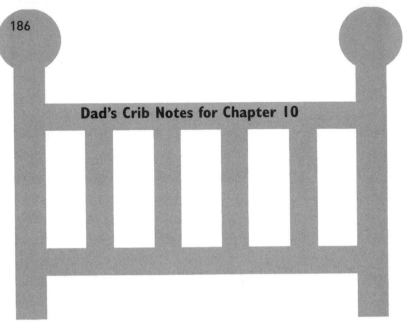

Dad's Crib Notes for Chapter 10

- In whatever time you have, try to squeeze in some quality bonding time with your child.
- It's important you begin building a strong relationship with your child right from the start.
- New fathers often have a difficult time finding where they fit in to the family. If you're feeling this way, make sure to talk to your BMP.
- Your partner will be the main decider in the debate of bottle-feeding versus breastfeeding, but be informed so the two of you can discuss it.
- Your child's grandparents can be a source of frustration for you and your BMP, but they tend to be especially kind to their grandchildren. This makes them ideal babysitters!
- This new baby is going to affect your schedule dramatically, so be ready to feel tired.
- It will take time for this adjustment, as with everything, from getting back to work to your sex life with your BMP. Just remember: everything in good time.

- Just as you researched your type of crib, health-care providers, and even your day care, now do a little research to find an ideal babysitter for your baby.
- Babyproofing your house before your child becomes mobile is an important safety step. Infants love to stick anything and everything in their mouth.

Doughnuts for Dad

My youngest daughter of three is beginning her education, and my wife alerted me to a flyer that was sent home concerning "Doughnuts for Dads," a program that was to begin at 8 A.M. I felt some frustration because I had to get in to work that day to deal with some issues that had come up, but I didn't want to disappoint my daughter. I hoped it would last just a few minutes. Perhaps I could pick up a free doughnut and chug some coffee, give my daughter a kiss, and be on my way.

When I got there, I got wind of the fact that they had a little program planned for the dads. In all honesty, my only thought was the delay this was going to cause. The program consisted of mad-lib-style poems they had written with their teacher's help, the title of which was, "My Amazing Dad." The first couple of kids came and went and there were a few laughs to be had. When it came my daughter's turn, my attitude about everything that was going on that morning completely changed.

I learned that my daughter thinks I am the best dad in the whole world because I play with her. I discovered my

189

favorite color is purple (it isn't) and that my favorite foods are "waffles and pancakes" (they aren't, but I often make weekend breakfast). I discovered I am "as strong as food." While everyone including me got a chuckle, I knew what she meant because I'm always telling her food will make her grow big and strong. She wishes we could play every day. She wrote her own name at the bottom of the story. To say that her story meant a lot to me would not sufficiently describe it. I felt so proud of her, and so happy that I was lucky enough to be her dad. Needless to say, I check from time to time to see when the next father's event is to be held. I wouldn't miss it for the world.

A Real Birth Story

Up until this point, we've focused mostly on the what and how of pregnancy. How to pick a doctor, what to do if there are complications, how manipulative grandparents wear you down so as to get their severely wrinkled hands on their grandchild. But one thing we haven't spent too much time on is the actual birth. What are some of the thoughts and feelings going on while all of this medical terminology springs to life? Is it really going to look like the birthing class video? Can I man up and cut the umbilical cord? So what we are going to do here is take you through a real pregnancy situation and birth, told through the eyes of the father.

It was springtime in the South, and not even the pine pollen could take away from my nervous excitement. My wife was pregnant, and we were closing in on the due date. Tall and skinny, my beautiful wife looked like a sporty car with one of those big travel "eggs" strapped onto her. Boy, that baby looked big in there! We knew it was going to be a girl because we simply could not resist finding out the sex of the baby. We had considered keeping it a surprise, but when it came down to it, and the ultrasound technician asked, since she was already looking, "Did you want to know?" we took the plunge.

We had a name selected, but it was being closely protected from prying family. To be honest, we didn't really want their feedback, positive or otherwise. We had the name suggestion box, and after reading the groups of names that had been scribbled on paper and dropped in, we were not sure whose taste we could trust anymore.

Then, as we were in the last few weeks approaching the due date, we went in to a doctor's appointment thinking we were on track. Only, at this appointment we discovered that our baby had become breech. [Author's Note: Breech babies are turned the wrong way for delivery. See, you learned something new today.] Because everything had gone relatively smoothly to this point, we weren't quite sure what to do. Our patient doctor covered the problems a breech baby can present and explained that they would attempt a "version." [Author's Note: It's me again. This is a technique in which the doctor attempts to turn the baby the correct way. It works about 50 percent of the time.] If the baby remained breech, the doctor informed us, she might be deliverable this way, but sometimes a C-section is performed.

So we were back the next appointment, full of nerves and concern. We were really coming down to the wire on the due date! As the doctors came in, we weren't sure what to expect. I don't know what I was expecting, but I saw them use some sort of technique that, in reality, looked like they were just pressing on my wife's abdomen and forcing the baby to turn the correct way. Of course there's no way I would have tried to do it. After a few minutes of this we found out it was a success. Our child was turned to the correct delivery position and we were able to put all of those other possibilities out of our mind.

Now we were closing in on week 40. As excited as I felt, my wife was feeling ready to give birth. I could really tell the baby was wearing her out. At the same time, I knew she would carry the baby for another year if that was what was required of her. She was feeling that if the baby was ready, so was she. On the elevator on the way up to the doctor's office, she hinted that if there was a way to get a discussion started around inducing labor that she would be okay with that.

Once we were in the office, the doctor checked on my wife and the baby. I forget the exact conversation, but basically because we were so close to the due date, our doctor asked us about the possibility of induction. Seeing an opening, we basically told him that if he thought it was prudent, then we were quite okay with getting this delivery on the road.

For some reason, I figured this was a scheduled delivery, like one of the many (many!) doctor's appointments we had been to during the pregnancy. So you can imagine my surprise when we were told that this was more of an on-call situation. Once we got to thinking about it, it made more sense to us. The hospital of course needed to take care of those who had no choice but to deliver (because the baby had the final say on timing), and then take on the voluntary cases like ours. So we had an approximate date and time, but we were told to go about our routine and they would let us know.

So, we did go about our business. But throughout the day, we kept glancing at our cell phones. Are these things on? Are we sure they still work? Are they charged? And then as soon as we sat down to eat at our church's fish-fry dinner, the phone magically rang. It was the hospital. They were ready for us. There was no need to rush, they assured us, just get our belongings and head their way. Well, we felt strange finishing our meal, but knowing what we were about to do, we did it with a smile. We couldn't resist telling the people sitting at our table what was going on. They all wished us well, and we proceeded to get our things.

On the way to the hospital, it was exciting but slightly strange. After all the thoughts of rushing to the hospital, with Baby coming at any second, this was rather calm. We didn't need to run any red lights, didn't even worry about flooring the gas pedal when we saw a green light turn yellow. We talked. She was glad that she was going to be delivering soon, and we were both excited.

The staff at the hospital got us checked into our room. Northside Hospital in Atlanta is an award-winning facility that delivers over 18,000 babies a year. Based on its reputation, our tour, and the group of doctors we were working with, we felt that we were in good hands.

Our room was exactly the same as we saw on our tour. It almost looked like a normal bedroom. The bed of course was a hospital bed, and you couldn't help but notice the monitoring equipment that was present. But there was also a TV and movie player, and a music player, and it had a nice overall feel to it. I did see the small couch I would be sleeping on the next few nights, and I think my mind was playing tricks on me, because my back was starting to hurt already.

Once we found out that Dr. X [Author's Note: Name omitted for obvious reasons] was on call that evening, we were slightly disappointed. We had ranked the doctors in the group; she was not our top choice. She came by to say a brief hello, and then she was gone. The nursing staff continued our preparation. There were IVs to hook up, and the fetal monitoring belt. They assured us they would be able to keep an eye on the fetal monitor from the nurses' station. Then it was just the two of us. We talked and watched movies. The whole thing seemed, I don't know, calmer than what I had pictured.

As we waited for the Pitocin to work its magic, I could tell my wife was starting to feel labor pains. She was a trooper about the whole thing, but I could tell she was hurting. They couldn't give her the painkilling epidural right away. She was allowed ice chips to stay hydrated and that was about it.

We had a few moments of excitement. The fetal monitoring belt slipped out of place, and the nurses came pretty quickly. At least it was good to know someone was paying attention! There were moments when the baby's heart began going both faster and slower, and as a nervous first-timer, I was scared by both situations. Occasionally a nurse would stop by and check on us. I'm guessing we were a reasonable garden-variety delivery at this point. This seemed strange to me, as my child's birth seemed anything but normal to me.

Finally it began. The contractions finally warmed up and began to strengthen. I was amazed at the casual atmosphere surrounding these events. It was very matter-of-fact as my wife began to push out our child. Nurses hovered, family was in the waiting area (hopefully to stay), and this dad was nervous. I felt excited and jumpy, both scared something was going to go wrong and excited that nothing seemed wrong at the moment.

Just when it seemed the doctor was going to miss all of the fun, she showed up. I had really been hoping she was going to make an appearance. The baby's head was already starting to show (look at that hair!), and I was considering either yelling for help or putting on those gloves—I couldn't decide. The doctor showed up, and the whole thing was pretty quick from that point. All of a sudden, "WHOOSH!" the baby was out, and the doctor was offering me the honor of cutting the umbilical cord. I declined, partly because of being slightly squeamish around blood and partly because I was scared I would mess up and injure my child in some way.

As quickly as it had started, it was over. The doctor was gone like a flash, and the nurses took it from there. They took our beautiful baby girl under the heat lamp, and checked her out, For some reason I wanted her to get a perfect score on the Apgar test. They assured us everything was in good order, and we could hold the baby. We took turns for a minute before unleashing the grandparents on the poor child. We were moved pretty quickly from the delivery room to the recovery room, and my father-in-law was kind enough to help us celebrate by sparing us the cafeteria and getting us some great food.

In the recovery room, we were all smiles. The nurses came in and attached matching bracelets to Mom, Dad, and Baby so there would be no doubt which baby belonged to us. They also told us that an alarm would go off if our child was taken past a certain point in the hospital. Scary thought!

Once we settled into our recovery room, we learned about how things would go for the next few days. The nurses would be happy to watch our girl in the nursery for us, and we could come get her at any time. When we had her, there was a panic button available for us if something went wrong. As for us, we had a TV, but all of our conversation and attention was on our baby. We felt like we should keep her with us as much as possible. I know, despite what the nurses said, I felt if I sent her to the nursery I would already be shirking my duty as a dad!

So keep her we did. One of us always tried to stay awake to make sure she was okay and breathing. It's something I thought was just us, but it seems all new parents do it: we're so scared something is going to happen that we listen to our babies breathe. Once at somewhere around 3 A.M. the nurse finally convinced me I should let our newborn go to the nursery and the parents should get some sleep. It was hard for me to refuse, because I was asleep holding my daughter anyway.

The only other excitement came when our daughter began coughing, and then began, as far as we could tell, choking. We looked at each other for what felt like forever, and then my wife smashed the panic button. A nurse came storming into our rooms, with urgency, but with the confidence of someone who knows what she is doing. While my wife told her our daughter was choking, I just sat there, pointing at the baby and saying, "choking!" The nurse simply nodded, gently but firmly took our child, flipped her over, and gave her a few well-placed thuds on the back. Whatever it was clogging things up was released, and all was well with the world again. The nurse, now one of my favorite people in the world, calmly left, and on her way out she told us to notify them if it happened again.

Now that the excitement was over, I took a deep breath. We felt like maybe our one scare was over. We decided to let our daughter spend a little more time in the nursery during the rest of our stay as we figured there was nowhere she would be safer. The rest of our visit was actually nice. We had a lot of time just to enjoy our child and share some time together.

As we left the hospital, we were a little sad. We knew we were reentering the real world. As I pulled the car around, we double-checked the infant car seat to make sure it was secure, and then we triple-checked to see whether we had buckled her in correctly. On the way home, we couldn't help but check on her constantly. It felt good to bring her home to her home, and to the room we had redone for her. We knew it was the start of a different phase of our lives together.

Told with the permission of John Mueller

Pretty cool, huh? This narrative was a father's account of the birth of his daughter, told in his words. As you can see, giving birth comes at you fast. That's why birth plans became both so popular and elaborate, because there isn't time for careful consideration and research when problems arise. Those decisions need to be already researched and discussed, and options evaluated by the time your bundle of joy enters your life.

Additional Resources

As much as it pains me to put this into print, I will tell you something my wife figured out a long time ago: I don't know everything. Because this topic is as old as people themselves, there is a lot written on the subject matter, of course. There are circumstances that may arise during the pregnancy where you may need to drill down deeper into certain subject matter. Pregnancy has been covered by many people in many styles from mild to wild, and everywhere in between. Because the styles and manner in which the information is presented and prioritized, it is helpful to gain multiple perspectives on this topic.

I wouldn't be paying homage to the era of lawyers if I didn't tell you that these are sources of information I recommend, but by all means, direct specific questions to your chosen health-care provider. They are the ones with the malpractice insurance after all. So depending on your needs, here are ten of the most helpful resources I have discovered:

What to Expect When You're Expecting
(Heidi Murkoff, Sharon Mazel)
This is roughly the equivalent of the Bible for members of the Christian faith. Lots of juicy and well researched information lies within these pages. Plus you can review yet another "For Dads" section written by, wait for it, a woman. But lots of the detailed medical stuff is spot-on. Special tip:

the real good stuff by Dads for Dads is on the website of the same name in the "Message Board" area.

Webmd.com

All the information is there for you to go ahead and misdiagnose your situation. So go ahead, tell me you're not confused by the article saying your child's ADHD could just be immaturity. Which one is it? But seriously, there's tons of useful information here for you.

About.com

They have so much here, especially in the "Men's Health" section. Remember when we were discussing you taking care of yourself? This site has a good bit of helpful information to that end.

Nelson DeMille

What does Mr. DeMille have to do with pregnancy? Nothing, to be honest. But between all of the doctor's appointments and potential waiting to be done, I suggest you keep a good book around to help pass the time. Anything John Corey especially.

PregnancyGuideOnline.com

It's an easy-to-reference website where the links for each week are right there for you in a bold purple. As you click into the respective weeks, try to stay focused on the useful information and not be distracted by the avant-garde cartoons of your BMP's insides.

Mayoclinic.com

Quick, you need medical advice! Where do you turn? For my two cents, the Mayo Clinic seems like a trustworthy source. Although not on par with *The Onion* as far as entertainment value, if you need accurate medical advice this is your go-to.

Paternityangel.com

This is a good website written from a man's perspective. The articles and lists are topical and informative as well.

Babynames.com

We got you started in Chapter 5, but of course you are going to want to consider every possible name combination. This site is a good place to start, with everything from the general lists of popular names to ones like "Popular baby names in Germany."

BabiesRUs.com

It's the Wal-Mart of baby stores. But boy do they have selection. It always pays to shop around, but this is a good place to get an idea as to what exactly is out there.

Babycenter.com

This well organized and informational website has lots of great articles, especially on selecting an obstetrician.

INDEX

DAILY BENDER

Want Some More?

Hit up our humor blog, The Daily Bender, to get your fill of all things funny—be it subversive, odd, offbeat, or just plain mean. The Bender editors are there to get you through the day and on your way to happy hour. Whether we're linking to the latest video that made us laugh or calling out (or bullshit on) whatever's happening, we've got what you need for a good laugh.

If you like our book, you'll love our blog. (And if you hated it, "man up" and tell us why.) Visit The Daily Bender for a shot of humor that'll serve you until the bartender can.

Sign up for our newsletter at

www.adamsmedia.com/blog/humor

and download our Top Ten Maxims No Man Should Live Without.

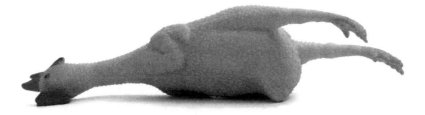

About the Author

John Pfeiffer is a financial advisor, author, and married father of three girls. He thought he met "the one" at least 300 times, but always ended up being disappointed . . . until he met her.

"Her" came with a mini-her in the form of a soon-to-be stepdaughter, which allowed Pfeiffer to perfect his parenting skills before his wife became pregnant with their first child. Since nothing horrible happened to either child over the next few years (mostly because of his wife's watchful eye), they decided to give it one more go—this time with the help of a third party. (Pfeiffer thought threesome; his wife corrected: fertility doctor.)

The fertility doctor was able to introduce an aggressive sperm cell to a receptive egg, and they had their third and final bundle o' joy. So as the father of a stepdaughter, a naturally conceived daughter, and a genetically enhanced superbaby, Pfeiffer is especially qualified to take expectant dads all the way through pregnancy's home stretch (pun intended).